Megan Arroll (PhD, C.Psychol., C.Sci., FHEA, AFBPsS) is a research fellow at the University of East London. She has been conducting research into medically unexplained and misunderstood illnesses for over a decade, and has published numerous academic papers on the topic of chronic fatigue syndrome/myalgic encephalomyelitis (CFS/ME). Megan is actively involved in a number of UK-based CFS/ME charities and patient organizations. She is the author of *Chronic Fatigue Syndrome: What you need to know about CFS/ME*, also published by Sheldon Press.

Christine P. Dancey (C.Psychol., C.Health Psychol., FHEA, FBPsS) is Emeritus Professor of Psychology at the University of East London. Christine has carried out research into chronic physical illness for over 25 years, and has written numerous publications in this field. She is a co-founder of the IBS Network, the only national IBS support group in the UK.

Megan and Christine have a close working relationship and are both members of the Chronic Illness Research Team based at the University of East London.

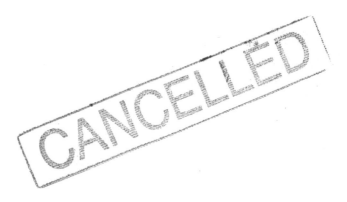

Overcoming Common Problems Series

Selected titles

A full list of titles is available from Sheldon Press,
36 Causton Street, London SW1P 4ST and on our website at
www.sheldonpress.co.uk

Overcoming Common Problems

Invisible Illness
Coping with misunderstood conditions

DR MEGAN A. ARROLL
and
PROFESSOR CHRISTINE P. DANCEY

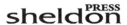

First published in Great Britain in 2014

Sheldon Press
36 Causton Street
London SW1P 4ST
www.sheldonpress.co.uk

British Library Cataloguing-in-Publication Data
A catalogue record for this book is available from the British Library

ISBN 978–1–84709–305–9
eBook ISBN 978–1–84709–306–6

Typeset by Caroline Waldron, Wirral, Cheshire
First printed in Great Britain by Ashford Colour Press
Subsequently digitally reprinted in Great Britain

eBook by Fakenham Prepress Solutions, Fakenham, Norfolk NR21 8NN

Produced on paper from sustainable forests

Contents

Megan would like to dedicate this book to everyone with an invisible illness. Both Christine and I know how tough it is when you look fine but are crippled with pain, fatigue, vertigo and a plethora of symptoms all at once. Your courage in the face of such debilitating symptoms is admirable. And of course thanks is given to my Ma, as always.

Christine would like to dedicate this book to Elisabeth Bond, who is one of the nicest and kindest people I have ever had the pleasure to know.

Foreword

This is an accessible and easy to read book for anyone affected by, or with an interest in, invisible illnesses. With no outward symptoms, invisible illnesses are often complex and misunderstood. They affect a great number of people and, for those who live with one of these conditions, they can be extremely debilitating and distressing; especially if their condition is not recognised or accepted.

At the Ménière's Society, we speak to people daily who have an invisible illness, 'I look fine on the outside, so how do I explain to someone that I'm not?' They want to know how to cope with their condition, to feel they are living a 'normal' life and know that they are not alone in their experience. These questions and anxieties are common to all invisible conditions and are addressed herein. As well as Ménière's disease, this book covers irritable bowel syndrome (IBS), migraine, fibromyalgia syndrome (FMS), chronic fatigue syndrome/myalgic encephalomyelitis (CFS/ME) and mal de débarquement syndrome (MdDS).

Dr Megan Arroll and Professor Christine Dancey's experience of invisible conditions comes from both an academic and personal background. They are both part of the University of East London's Chronic Illness Research Team, which has 20 years' experience studying various invisible illnesses, and have published widely on this topic. In addition, Christine and Megan have first-hand experience and understanding of invisible illnesses, including CFS/ME, interstitial cystitis, IBS and endometriosis. They know exactly how these conditions affect people, having been through them themselves. Here they share their knowledge and experience, along with the personal stories of others, to offer a valuable insight for the benefit of everyone affected by an invisible illness.

Drawing on clinical and personal experience, as well as recent research, this book gives an expert and personal insight into living with and managing an invisible illness; whether you have an invisible condition yourself, have a family or friend who is affected, or just want to know more about the subject. It contains a clear description of each condition and covers a wide-range of topics, including symptoms, diagnosis, relationships, home and work life, sleep problems, depression, anxiety, treatments and self-management techniques. Plus, helpful suggestions for communicating with and explaining the condition to others – who are often unaware exactly how a person is affected.

With its practical tips and tools this book aims to help give people more confidence and reduce the isolation and anxieties associated with these conditions and the impact they have on a person's day-to-day life. As well as practical methods for managing the condition, it also gives information on how to get and where to go for additional information and support from others who share your experience. Once you've read this book, you will no doubt find yourself returning to it again and again to dip into specific chapters as part of the management of your condition. A helpful and useful resource for all.

Natasha Harrington-Benton, MA
Director, Ménière's Society

Preface

Both of us are academics – health psychologists – who have worked in universities and carried out research into chronic physical illnesses. We have researched many different conditions, including irritable bowel syndrome (IBS), inflammatory bowel disease, myalgic encephalomyelitis (ME), known as chronic fatigue syndrome (CFS), and mal de débarquement syndrome (MdDS). The illnesses we have focused on during our careers have tended to be invisible (ones where other people cannot tell you are ill unless you tell them). They also tend to be ones that are contested or misunderstood by health professionals and the general public, such as IBS. Researching these illnesses and finding out how they affect day-to-day lives is important for the person who has the illness and important for health professionals and other people who come into contact with those who are ill.

When we first began research into IBS in 1991, there was no national IBS organization and no self-help groups. The few research studies carried out into IBS tended to focus on the causes of IBS. This is important of course, but this type of research wasn't read by nurses and the general public, and so most people had no knowledge of IBS, and someone with IBS was unlikely to know anyone else with IBS. Thus a person with IBS at that time was likely to feel alone and isolated and to have little knowledge of the condition. We know this because we carried out research into the views and feelings of the patients themselves. Until this research, no one had published papers based on the views of people with IBS. Things are different now – there are lots of studies, many based on accounts given by people with the condition. So this book is based on research that we have carried out and on research from other people.

But we don't want you to think that we are stuffy academics who have no personal knowledge of these conditions. Unfortunately, we have.

Christine suffered from abdominal pains and bowel problems for at least seven years before she obtained a university post that had private medical insurance at reduced cost. For these seven years, during which she was a patient of the NHS in London, she saw many doctors and was admitted to hospital two or three times. She was always told she had IBS. As she became worse and worse, the diagnosis did not change, despite Christine complaining of additional symptoms that did not match those of IBS – terrible period pains, which were very irregular, and other more embarrassing symptoms, which even now she cannot bear to mention. She was told that these additional symptoms were the result of stress. To cut a very long story short, she got herself referred privately to a gynaecologist. A laparoscopy found stage 4 endometriosis. The bladder and the bowel were attached to the womb by adhesions. As the endometriosis was not caught in time, she was unable to have children. After hormone treatment she had a full hysterectomy. When Christine told her NHS doctors about this, they maintained that she had both IBS and endometriosis. After correct treatment for endometriosis, Christine never again suffered from 'IBS symptoms'. Although Christine is really bad at remembering people's names, she has never forgotten the consultant who, on hearing her symptoms, immediately said he thought they were due to endometriosis, and gave her back her life.

Fast-forward 16 years: Christine was laid low with a viral illness – a very high temperature, aches and pains, extreme tiredness. By this time Christine had moved to Suffolk, where the NHS doctors in her area were known to be really good, and they were. They immediately referred her to specialists. Various blood tests showed abnormalities, and the pattern of results indicated a viral infection. She was told she was unlikely to get back to work for three or four weeks. Blood results were monitored regularly, and each time the tests still showed abnormalities, although over time the results became less abnormal. Christine couldn't walk, had no appetite and was totally exhausted. For the first few months she slept well at night and also slept during the day. Then the pattern changed and she found she couldn't sleep, often sleeping for just two hours a night. She couldn't bear light or any sort of noise. She couldn't read, watch TV or do anything much. She had to have help to get to the shower and bathroom. ME was provisionally diagnosed and later – much later – came a firm diagnosis from the specialists. Christine spent a year at home, and gradually recovered enough to go back to work. Christine felt supported by her doctors, who helped her during these very dark times. It's really important for people with chronic illness to have the support of their doctors. If your doctors are not supportive, we hope you will be able to change to ones who will support you.

Christine and Megan have many things in common and unfortunately having numerous contested illnesses is one of them! During Megan's childhood and her teenage years, she was very active indeed; she loved dancing and being outdoors and with her friends – the usual stuff of childhood, really. Then, at the age of 14 she came down with a virus and the tests showed it was glandular fever. She was quite sick for a number of weeks and was off school but began to recover, and by the end of the school term she felt quite well. Then during the summer holidays, Megan's health began to deteriorate. Much as with

Christine's experience, Megan could not stand any light or noise, had absolutely no energy and lost a great deal of weight, at one point weighing only 40 kilograms (six and a half stone). Megan's sensitivity to any sound or light was so great, she spent all her time in a darkened room, with the TV often being too much to bear. She vividly remembers that, inside, her mind was still OK, still active, but that communicating often took far too much energy. She was taken to the GP what felt like hundreds of times, and all the tests showed negative results. The GP then decided Megan was simply depressed and prescribed strong anti-depressants, which made her much, much worse. At the time, there was so little understanding that the school threatened to sue Megan's parents for non-attendance, and it wasn't until she saw an educational psychologist that there was any mention of the condition known as CFS/ME. It was a shock for her to read the associated information; everything fitted together.

However, there were (and still are to some extent) so few treatment options that simply, and finally, gaining a diagnosis was not the relief it appeared to be. Megan and her family tried everything, but the symptoms were starting to get even worse. So, the decision was made to stop and take the pressure off finding a magical cure. Gradually, so slowly that it wasn't even noticeable on a daily basis, Megan began to recover and was well enough to attend university in her late teens.

Sadly, this is not the only invisible illness Megan has experienced. After years of extremely painful bladder infections, Megan finally begged her doctor to tell her the name of a good urologist, even if it cost a fortune. She was then diagnosed with chronic bladder inflammation and interstitial cystitis. Although this is a long-term condition, treatment has helped enormously and diminished symptoms that had become so bad that Megan couldn't leave the house for fear of being more than a few yards away from a toilet. Recently, yet another battle has begun and, as in Christine's case, although doctors first attributed symptoms to IBS, it seems the culprit may be endometriosis.

The aim of these personal stories is not to gain any sort of sympathy, but rather to let you, the reader, know that we know how misunderstood conditions actually *feel*, physically, emotionally and socially. We have spent the majority of our research careers investigating these conditions and will continue to do so, in the hope that even if science doesn't give us more answers in the near future, at the very least we don't all need to hide and feel ashamed and isolated by our bodies that can, at times, seem like the enemy within.

(By the way, Christine and Megan also have other, more positive things in common – it's certainly not all doom and gloom! A great love for animals is one of them.)

Acknowledgements and note to the reader

We would like to give thanks to Elisabeth Bond, Cait Capp and Jo Johnstone for reading the draft manuscript and for giving suggestions for change; the book has been improved by all your input! We would also like to thank Natasha Harrington-Benton for kindly writing the foreword to the book and Shayne Town and Ann-Marie Loponen for providing us with their illustrations. Finally, we give a heartfelt thanks to Fiona Marshall, who worked with us to design this book for a wide range of readers; we have very much enjoyed working with you, Fiona!

Note to the reader

This is not a medical book and is not intended to replace advice from your doctor. Consult your pharmacist or doctor if you believe you have any of the symptoms described, and if you think you might need medical help.

1

Introduction to misunderstood illnesses

We must keep in mind that the whole human person – not merely a part of her brain – thinks, feels or believes. Indeed, the human person cannot be reduced to neural processes and it is difficult to understand a whole person without understanding the sociocultural context in which the person lives. Mind and brain are integrated and interdependent . . . the results of neuro-imaging studies strongly suggest that mentalistic variables (e.g. consciousness, metacognition, volition, beliefs, hopes) and their intentional content . . . are neither identical with nor reducible to brain processes.   (Beauregard, 2009, p. 14)

This chapter introduces you to the various illnesses covered in this book and shows the ways in which they can be described, such as acute or chronic, medically unexplained or explained, and common or rare. It also introduces you to the ways in which biological, psychological and social factors affect bodily systems such as the immune system, which can increase susceptibility to illness. In addition, it gives a brief introduction to what is known as the 'mind–brain–body problem' in relation to chronic illness.

Does the mind exist?

You know that your body exists (as you feel that 'you' inhabit your body), and you feel certain that your brain exists. You know that you can think and reason, and even though you cannot see your own brain, no doubt you have a good idea of what the brain looks like from books or TV programmes. However, whether the 'mind' exists is debatable.

It might seem odd to start a chapter on misunderstood illness with talk about the mind, but the mind is an essential concept in this book, as in very many other books on health and illness. There are many definitions of 'mind', which can easily be found in books and on the internet, and naturally these definitions differ. In this book we use the word 'mind' to mean what people (or animals) have that enables them to be aware of themselves and to think, feel, have intentions and carry out those intentions. If you decide to make a cup of tea now, who or what is making the decision? Is it your brain? Is it your mind? Do you 'make up your mind' to make a cup of tea, whereupon various neurones (nerve cells) in the brain fire up and carry out that intention? Or does your brain decide you want a cup of tea? Or are the brain and mind one and the same thing?

Does it matter?

Philosophers have debated whether the mind exists (as separate from the brain) for hundreds of years, and these discussions are very much alive today.

Some philosophers and psychologists believe that the mind is a by-product of the brain, or even that the mind is an illusion produced by the brain. The scientists who believe this believe that your brain is, essentially, *you*. These scientists are called materialists, and this view is called materialism. Many scientists (but not all) are materialists.

The quotation at the beginning of this chapter is by a scientist who is a non-materialist. Non-materialists believe that the mind and the brain are two different types of entities, although the mind and brain affect, and are affected by, each other. No one knows which view is correct, although many think they do. These are philosophical debates, which probably don't affect the average person going about his or her daily life. To all intents and purposes, people generally assume that they have free will, and that they control their lives. People act as if they have 'minds' and they talk about their 'minds' – for example, 'I made up my mind to see it through' or 'I'm going out of my mind!'

This book takes the view that the mind and brain are two different aspects of the whole person. This isn't because we have explored all the philosophical debates and have chosen this view, it's because we have read many articles relating to the ways in which psychological and social factors can influence illness, in particular, placebo studies and neuroimaging studies, which, to us, demonstrate that certain mind techniques, such as guided imagery, can affect the brain and the body. An example of a simple guided imagery exercise would be to ask people to visualize a calming experience – they might think about a favourite place, a garden or a beach. They might be asked to imagine walking through the garden, focusing on the colours, the calmness, the smell of the flowers and so on. There are many studies that show that guided imagery can lower pulse and heart rate. There are also some imagery exercises that can have beneficial results on the immune system.

The mind–brain–body in relation to illness

Even though we now know the mind, brain and body affect one another, people still talk about 'mental illness' and 'physical illness', whereas in reality all systems (the mind, the brain and the body) are involved in illness, whether the symptoms are primarily physical or non-physical.

The mind, brain and body systems work together. In fact all systems interact with one another – systems such as the nervous, endocrine (hormonal), digestive, respiratory, cardiovascular and immune systems. A relatively new field of study – the psychoneuroimmunology of illness and disease – looks at the way the body systems affect and are affected by psychosocial factors such as stress and depression, and by illness and disease. These factors can't be considered to be independent. For instance, we now know that both physical and psychosocial factors can trigger an immune response in the body, which can increase susceptibility to illness. Normally, the immune system aids in preventing disease and assisting in our recovery. It recognizes potentially harmful invaders such as viruses and bacteria. This allows the immune system to mount a response to get rid of these harmful agents. The main way the immune system does this is by using various types of cell. For example, cells called T lymphocytes can destroy or deactivate viruses and bacteria. There are also T-helper cells (which trigger the immune response), natural killer cells (which detect cells taken over by cancer or viruses and destroy them), and B cells (which manufacture antibodies). Detailed discussion of these cells is beyond the scope of this book, but we mention more about them in the chapters that follow.

The field of psychoneuroimmunology investigates a connection between psychological factors, changes in the immune system and changes in health. Years ago people thought the immune system was a closed system that didn't interact with the brain and nervous system, but more and more research has shown links between the immune system and the brain and behaviour. Stress and mentalistic variables such as depression, thoughts and feelings can all affect immunity. For instance, once you experience stress, your heart rate increases. As well as this, your endocrine system releases hormones in response to stress. The effects of brain processes and the immune system are bi-directional – both physical and psychosocial factors can affect the immune system, which in turn can cause illness or disease. This is supported by a wealth of scientific evidence. Influenza is caused by a virus (and viruses are certainly a 'physical' cause of illness), and it causes bodily symptoms, which we have all experienced. The effects of the virus on the body can cause depressed mood and mental fatigue as well as physical fatigue. Research shows that people who are stressed are more likely to be susceptible to flu than those who are not so stressed. Stress has harmful effects on the immune system and makes you more likely to become ill. Many psychological and social factors can influence the *progression* of a disease, even if these factors played no part in causing or triggering your disease. Psychoneuroimmunology shows that *you* can have some influence over the progression of your illness. The way you think about your illness affects not only your brain but also your body, and vice versa. This is good, because you will find that certain psychological techniques will help you to live with and cope with your illness, even if the symptoms remain.

Although it would be interesting to talk more about mind, brain and body, there are many books that cover these topics (see Further reading). However, the relationships between the mind, brain and body in relation to illness are mentioned in the chapters that follow.

Illnesses, diseases, disorders and conditions

The word 'illness' encompasses diseases, disorders and conditions. Illness is the experience you have when you are suffering from a disease, disorder, or condition.

Disease refers to an illness in which there is medical evidence of a disease process. Examples are cancer, where tumours may be apparent, or ulcers and inflammation of the colon, as in inflammatory bowel disease (which is an umbrella term for ulcerative colitis and Crohn's disease). Many diseases tend to become worse over time unless treated, and may sometimes be fatal. These diseases are legitimized (accepted as 'real') by the medical profession because there is medical evidence that the body is diseased, and patients with such diseases are treated seriously. Often (although not always) the cause or causes of diseases are known and there are clear criteria for diagnosis, and treatments are available, although these treatments are not always fully successful. People tend to think of these diseases as purely physical – that is, they consider that psychological and social factors do not cause, aggravate or trigger the disease.

There are thousands of illnesses. These vary from the very common, such as IBS, which affects millions of people world-wide, to the extremely rare, some of which affect only a few families. (These are usually genetic diseases.) An illness is defined as rare in Europe when it affects fewer than 1 in 2,000 people, whereas in the USA an illness is defined as rare when it affects fewer than 200,000 individuals at any given time (see http://www.rarediseaseday.org). There are between 6,000 and 8,000 rare diseases worldwide.

Most of the illnesses in this book do not have the status of 'disease'. An example is IBS. Experts disagree on the cause or causes of illnesses such as IBS. Although the symptoms may vary in frequency and severity, over time people with IBS, on average, do not tend to get worse. Illnesses such as these are called 'functional' because the problem seems to be a fault in the way the body system works (in this case the gastrointestinal system), rather than the symptoms being due to an actual disease process. So we do not say 'irritable bowel disease', since we haven't got evidence of a disease process. Instead, we tend to say IBS is a condition or a disorder. People often use these terms interchangeably. (In fact, in an article from 2013 in the journal *Biomedical Scientist*, experts stated that 'IBS and IBD are the two gastrointestinal *diseases* [our emphasis] that are most similar'.

Some people (often psychiatrists) have concluded that psychological processes directly cause the symptoms of illnesses such as these. This is likely to be because:

- there is no medical evidence of a disease process (yet!);
- the symptoms are variable, both in frequency and severity;
- people with these illnesses often have high levels of depression and anxiety.

However, stating that psychological processes can directly cause illnesses such as these is too simplistic – it is more complicated than this, as you will see in the following chapters.

Acute and chronic illness

Acute illnesses come on suddenly, and last a short time. These illnesses tend to have known symptoms, which are much the same for everyone. A cold or flu are examples. Such illnesses are often caused by viruses or bacteria, and are often self-limiting, so that people often get better without any medical intervention. Heart attacks and strokes are acute illnesses that are obviously not self-limiting; medical treatment is needed quickly. Acute illnesses like these come on suddenly, although there may be long-lasting effects.

Chronic illnesses, by definition, last over time – diabetes, arthritis, and IBS and the other illnesses in this book are examples of chronic illnesses. How long a chronic illness lasts varies, and there can be vast differences between people. For example, some people with IBS see an improvement within a year, whereas others might have IBS for 20 or more years. The average duration of CFS/ME is three years, but again some people improve within one year, and a minority of people have symptoms for over 20 years.

Medically unexplained or contested disorders (MUDs, probably as in 'as clear as mud')

CFS/ME and IBS are examples of medically unexplained disorders (or MUDs), and are sometimes called 'contested disorders'. They are medically unexplained because we don't know exactly what causes them, and they are contested because different 'experts' have different views as to the causes. However, there have been illnesses in the past labelled as 'psychosomatic' or 'psychological' that are now recognized as having a known medical cause. Illnesses that cannot be explained by a disease process may be labelled in this way. At one time Parkinson's disease was explained as psychosomatic, schizophrenia was supposed to be caused by emotionally cold mothers, and stomach ulcers were said to be caused by stress. These explanations are now discredited.

These types of illness tend to be misunderstood, by both health professionals and the general public. A lack of knowledge often means that those affected are not given the understanding and support they need. When we first started research into IBS in 1991, we found that many people with IBS knew no one else with the same condition, and tried to hide their illnesses from others. They often felt ashamed, and blamed themselves for their symptoms. When we lectured about IBS to students, ripples of laughter would sweep through the lecture hall, as we talked about diarrhoea and constipation. People did not take IBS seriously. When the first book about IBS was published, one medical practitioner said that he was surprised that someone could write more about IBS than would fit into a leaflet! Now, we can lecture to students about IBS feeling fairly confident that they will not laugh – most know friends or relatives with IBS, and some have it themselves. Many students now are happy to relate details of their illness to us and will often speak in class about it.

The stigma attached to IBS has decreased over the years. Over the past 20 years, self-help groups and organizations for people with IBS (and medical professionals) have helped to bring knowledge of this disorder to health professionals, the general public and of course people with IBS. People with the disorder might have the same severity and frequency of symptoms as they had previously, but many now have a wide knowledge about IBS and no longer feel the need to hide their condition. Not feeling so stigmatized, being able to talk about their illness and feeling confident that most people will take it seriously makes it easier for them to manage their condition.

Contested or medically unexplained disorders are difficult for health professionals to deal with. By definition, there is no disease process to account for the symptoms and, with no known cause, there is no treatment that has lasting effects for everyone with the disorder. Health professionals can become frustrated when treatments don't work.

Indeed, health professionals sometimes do not seem to know much about certain disorders. People have been told that their illness is most likely due to stress and are simply told to reduce it. Other professionals doubt that a disorder is real because it cannot be seen. We were told (by a health psychologist who should have known better) that 'there is no such thing as ME'. Others denigrate it by talking as if having CFS/ME is just like being extremely tired and something you should be able to deal with. When one person told an acquaintance that she had CSF/ME, he replied, 'Oh, that's just feeling tired all the time, isn't it?' These attitudes matter because research shows that people who have an illness that is not legitimized and taken seriously by others are more anxious and depressed than people with similar symptoms but whose illness is legitimized.

Misunderstood illnesses

There are numerous illnesses that we could have focused on in this book. Although we mention other illnesses to illustrate certain points, our main focus is on the chronic physical illnesses that have tended to be misunderstood or trivialized, and how you can cope with these illnesses.

To be quite open about our approach: we do not believe that psychological factors can by themselves *cause* diseases and illnesses. However, our research over more than 20 years has led us to believe that psychosocial factors can *interact* with physical and medical factors to trigger relapses or worsen illnesses. We know, again from the research, that certain psychosocial factors can *influence the progress* of the illness. This is a good thing, because it means that you will be able to manage your illness more effectively. Your symptoms may remain, but they will become less intrusive, and you will be able to cope better. It is not easy to do this, but it is worth it. Although we make brief mention of some of these techniques in Chapters 1–5, we focus on them in Chapters 6 and 7.

The illnesses that we are focus on in this book are:

- irritable bowel syndrome (IBS)
- migraine

IBS – THE DIALOGUE

IBS – THE SUB-TEXT

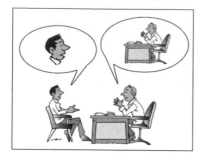

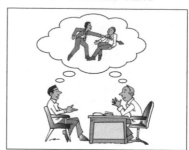

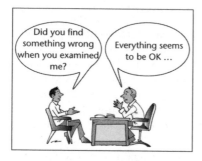

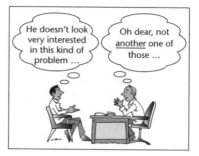

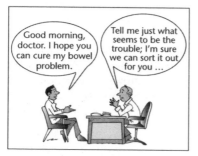

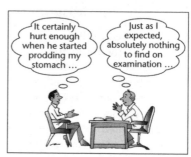

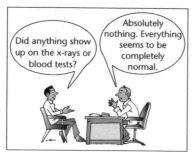

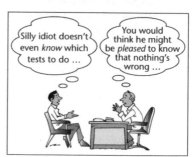

IBS – THE DIALOGUE

IBS – THE SUB-TEXT

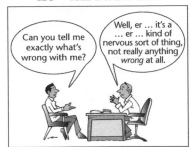

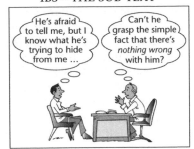

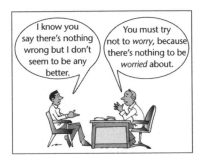

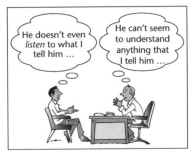

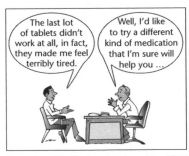

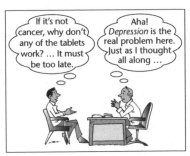

Reproduced by kind permission of David Wingate.

- fibromyalgia syndrome (FMS)
- chronic fatigue syndrome/ myalgic encephalomyelitis (CFS/ME)
- Ménière's disease
- Mal de débarquement syndrome (MdDS).

IBS, FMS, CFS/ME and migraine are invisible chronic illnesses that affect hundreds of thousands of people world-wide, and IBS, FMS and CFS/ME are contested disorders. Recently migraine has been found to have a large genetic component to it. MdDS ('mal de débarquement' is

French for 'disembarkation sickness') is a neurological condition that affects some people after being on transport, usually a boat or a ship, for a long time. People for whom MdDS started after disembarking from a ship, for example, still feel as if they are on a ship, bobbing and rocking around, even though they are on dry land. This is, of course, very debilitating. It is a rare disorder, and a medical practitioner is unlikely ever to have seen a patient with it.

Ménière's disease is of course defined as a disease; it is chronic, but it is invisible to others and has unpredictable symptoms, such as attacks of vertigo, that are often misunderstood. (Vertigo is a dizzying symptom whereby someone feels as if the room or environment is spinning around. This sensation is often accompanied by nausea and sickness. In migraine this is due to dysfunction of the vestibular (balance) system.)

These illnesses are described in detail in Chapter 2. The conditions in this book vary in the extent to which they are misunderstood and legitimized by others and in the frequency, severity and predictability of their symptoms. They are often invisible to others, and unless the person chooses to disclose the condition or the symptoms become apparent – such as a sudden vertigo attack in public, although even here people may just believe the affected person is drunk – a person with one of these illnesses may seem perfectly well.

Looking well when you are feeling dreadful has disadvantages. People with invisible chronic illness have been accused of being lazy or malingering. Taking time off work when you look well leads to suspicions that you are not really ill. People can give sympathy to people who are obviously disabled but are less likely to be sympathetic to those who look fine. For instance, standing in one place tends to be difficult for people with CFS/ME. Thus queuing can be problematic. For people with IBS, queuing for the toilet might be a problem. Many people with chronic illnesses find it difficult to ask others for help. In the UK, CFS/ME and IBS organizations give cards to their members, which they can show to others to get help. Letters to these organizations show that while some people have received help, such as letting them go to the front the queue, others have found that people have not been at all helpful (this is our tactful way of putting it).

Having a chronic illness changes your life, and in order to cope and maintain some sense of equilibrium, you have to adapt, both to your symptoms and the perception of yourself as an ill or disabled person. Particularly with a medically unexplained illness, you may have to spend some time discovering all there is to know about the disorder. This can be difficult. For instance, when Sue Backhouse and Christine Dancey first set up the IBS Network (UK) in 1991, there was only one book on IBS for the layperson, and many people had not heard of the condition. At that time, there was no UK organization for people with IBS and there were no self-help groups. People with illnesses that have unpredictable or embarrassing symptoms are more likely to feel a loss of control, which can lead to depression and helplessness.

When Jane Houghton first experienced MdDS, nobody knew what was wrong with her. Jane researched her condition through the internet and found the MdDS USA website. There was no UK self-help group and most medical practitioners had never heard of the condition. Jane had to find out as much information as she could about MdDS, and she had to adapt to living with MdDS and to try to find a way to cope with the condition. Jane now spends much of her time publicizing MdDS (see <http://www.mdds.org.uk>).

As psychologists, we can't give you medical advice on your illness. You need to become an expert in your own illness and have an open mind towards techniques that may or may not work. We have found that people with a physical chronic illness often dismiss any discussion of the role of psychosocial factors in illness and disease. Just because your illness or disease might have a physical cause doesn't mean that psychological and social factors don't matter.

Summary and conclusion

In this chapter we have introduced you to the illnesses that we concentrate on in this book. We have shown you that these misunderstood illnesses have many similarities, even though the symptoms and people's experiences of the illnesses may be very different. We have also shown that biological, psychological and social factors may influence certain aspects of these illnesses. In the chapters that follow, we discuss the role of biological, physiological and psychosocial factors in long-term illness. To recover, even partially, from an illness you need to have helpful psychosocial factors, as well as good treatment, good nutrition and friends. It is certainly worth working on your mind as well as your body. We hope this book helps you to do this.

2

Common invisible and misunderstood conditions

In all those years no one had recognized these symptoms; I was completely alone with this condition. I had recounted this story dozens of times only to receive baffled looks of 'how weird' from health professionals. Then, one day in my early 40s, when describing the symptoms to an occupational health nurse during a routine check-up, she said, 'What an extraordinary story! Oh, have you ever heard of disembarkation syndrome?' No, never, but now, after 30 years, I was on to something at last.

(CL, with MdDS)

This chapter outlines a number of conditions that we have researched and which have been found to have many things in common. A summary of each condition is presented, followed by a discussion of the similarities of the conditions in terms of origin, symptoms and diagnosis, how acute illnesses can become long-term conditions, and theories about why a greater proportion of women than men become ill with these conditions.

Irritable bowel syndrome (IBS)

Of all the conditions in this book, IBS is the most common, affecting between 15 and 22 per cent of people in Western societies. As with all the illnesses covered here, more women than men appear to have the symptoms of IBS. No one knows exactly why this is; there are theories suggesting that hormones, the way women respond physiologically to stress and also the way in which doctors diagnose conditions that are not associated with a disease process may influence how many men and women are diagnosed with IBS and other medically unexplained disorders.

If you have IBS, your symptoms may include:

- abdominal pain;
- change in bowel habits, such as diarrhoea or constipation – the change is important because what may be 'normal' for one person

may not be for another, and so comparing bowel habits with friends and family is not a very good measure of symptoms;

- urgency to have a bowel movement, which may include a feeling that the bowels have not emptied fully;
- flatulence;
- bloating;
- burbulence (rumblings and grumblings in the digestive system).

Symptoms tend to vary over time and from person to person, and it can often be difficult to spot a pattern. However, doctors should conduct a number of blood tests to rule out infections and other possible causes of abdominal discomfort.

If your doctor doesn't do any blood tests, you are within your rights to ask for these, as IBS symptoms are very similar to those of coeliac disease. Coeliac disease is caused by an autoimmune reaction to gluten, and this can easily be ruled out by a simple blood test. (As with all invisible illnesses, it is very important to exclude any condition that may be treatable, so do ensure that your doctor tests you for coeliac disease if you have the symptoms of IBS.) Gluten is a protein found in cereals (wheat, barley and rye); in coeliac disease the immune system mistakes gluten as a threat and then produces an immune response. During this response, the villi in the small intestine (tiny tube-shaped growths that help to digest food) are damaged, and this is what produces symptoms. There is no cure for coeliac disease, but a gluten-free diet can often resolve symptoms. People with IBS sometimes try a gluten-free diet as well but, at present, there is no consistent evidence that this is a useful treatment and it can be very difficult indeed to stay completely gluten-free.

However, diet can be a very important aspect in the management of some, but not all, symptoms of IBS. For people whose main symptom is diarrhoea, reducing insoluble fibre (fibre that cannot be digested but passes through the bowel) can help. Foods containing insoluble fibre include bran, wholegrain breads, cereals and nuts and seeds. People who suffer more from constipation may benefit from an increased intake of foods high in soluble fibre. Examples of these foods are bananas, apples, root vegetables, rye, barley and oats. Also increasing the volume of water that is consumed can help digestive transit (the movement of food through the digestive system). We will look more at treatments such as exercise, further dietary measures, stress reduction, probiotics and medication in Chapter 6.

Migraine

I drove down from London to visit my son near Southampton where he was on a work placement and lodging with a family. The journey itself was fairly stressful as I had only been there once before and I wasn't sure of the way. Having got there, we decided to go out for a pub lunch. As it was a treat for me, I had a glass of cider! I ate more than I usually do at lunchtime but I enjoyed it. Then we decided to take the ferry across the river to Southampton. The ferry smelt of oil or diesel fumes and it was difficult to look at the water because of the strong sunlight reflecting on it. By the time we had walked around Southampton for a while I felt the beginnings of a migraine. I didn't have any painkillers with me, stupidly enough. So by the time we got back to his lodgings I had started to feel nauseous and my head was thumping. I just felt like going to bed but couldn't do this in a stranger's house. So I said goodbye to my son and drove off. I knew that my friend's aunt Winnie lived nearby and thought I would see if she was in. I had only been there once before but I recognized the way to her house. Before I got there, however, I had to stop and throw up my wonderful lunch into a carrier bag, which was fortunately on the floor of the car. Finally I got to Winnie's house and rang the bell and, luckily for me, she was in. She was very calm as I lurched through the door asking if I could lie down on her bed. She didn't bat an eyelid at this unexpected visit from someone she barely knew and looked after me for the rest of the day until the next morning when I was able to leave. I felt washed out but much better. I've been eternally grateful to her for her impromptu hospitality. Looking back, I realized I had done everything a migraine sufferer shouldn't do. I shouldn't have drunk alcohol on an empty stomach, shouldn't have overeaten, and should have worn sunglasses and carried painkillers with me.

(JJ, with migraine)

Migraine is also relatively common, affecting approximately 18 per cent of women and 7 per cent of men in Western countries. People between the ages of 25 and 55 are the most likely to experience migraines, but this does not mean that other age groups are not affected as well. In fact, many people with migraine have their first attack when they are teenagers or children.

A migraine is not simply a bad headache; there are often many other symptoms during a migraine episode, which can differ between different people. Also, the pattern of migraine attacks can vary over time, similar to the symptoms of IBS above and other invisible conditions described below. A migraine is usually associated with throbbing on one side of the head, which gets worse with movement. Often when a migraine becomes full-blown, people need to lie down in a darkened room and keep very still.

Additional symptoms that can occur with a migraine include:

- nausea, which is sometimes followed by actual vomiting;
- increased sensitivity to light, sound and smells (known as photophobia, phonophobia and osmophobia, respectively);
- problems with concentration and attention (for example, it may be difficult to keep track of a conversation or follow a plot on the TV when normally this is not a problem at all);
- increased sweating for no external reason;
- feeling very hot or very cold;
- abdominal pain and sometimes diarrhoea;
- a frequent need to empty the bladder.

Not everyone has all these symptoms, and they may change from time to time in an individual. Somewhat surprisingly, these symptoms can occur *without* a headache and this can still be defined as a migraine. Symptoms tend to last anywhere from four hours to three days (sometimes longer) and can be severely disabling, affecting people's ability to work, to carry out their roles (as a mother, husband, carer) and to enjoy life.

One of the most characteristic features of a migraine is the aura, which is experienced by about a third of people who have migraines. The aura usually starts before the headache and pain, and it can be associated with:

- visual problems (some people can see flashing lights or zigzag patterns or have blind spots);
- bodily stiffness or a tingling sensation ('pins and needles'), usually in the neck, shoulders or limbs;
- difficulties with co-ordination (such as feeling disorientated or off-balance);
- problems speaking and finding the right words.

Aura symptoms are 'prodromal,' meaning that they can start between 15 minutes and one hour before the headache begins. But not everyone experiences an aura and some people get these sensations with only a mild headache or no headache at all.

Treatments for migraine include painkillers, other types of medication such as triptans, anti-inflammatory medications and anti-sickness medicines, hormonal treatments (for women who have a particular pattern of migraine associated with their menstrual cycle) and diet and lifestyle changes.

My migraines are generally around the temples and at the back of my head. Light hurts my eyes. I always want pressure applied to my head. Last month I had a slight migraine in the head but the nausea was overwhelming. I have once before suffered with blind spots in my vision. This lasted about five hours and once again was around the time of my period starting. I've suffered with migraines since adolescence. They have become progressively worse the older I have become. Thankfully I get them only once a month maybe for one to three days. This will always coincide with the one to three days before my period. Falling pregnant was great as I had no migraines for nine months plus for the eight months I breastfed my baby. I had forgotten how debilitating they were. However, I was soon reminded once they returned after I stopped breastfeeding. I have also noticed that many types of hormonal contraception bring on my migraines.   (SH, with migraine)

Fibromyalgia syndrome (FMS)

About 1 in 20 (or 5 per cent) of people throughout the world have symptoms that can be defined as FMS. Again, women are more likely than men to have FMS, and at least twice the number of women as men are diagnosed with this condition. People aged 30–60 represent the largest proportion of those with FMS, but it can also develop in children and older adults. As with IBS and migraine, there is no specific test for FMS and it can be difficult for doctors to diagnose. The symptoms of FMS come under these main headings:

- pain (aching, burning and/or stabbing sensations);
- extreme sensitivity, which includes 'hyperalgesia' (heightened sensitivity to pain) and 'allodynia' (when something that should not be painful at all, such as a very light touch, causes pain);
- stiffness, which is often severe after being in the same position for an extended period of time, such as on waking in the morning;
- fatigue, which is sometimes flu-like and often so severe that everyday activities are affected;
- sleep disturbance, such as non-restorative sleep, in which a person can sleep for a long period of time but not feel refreshed, possibly from not experiencing 'deep sleep';
- cognitive difficulties, such as problems with remembering or learning new information, problems in concentrating, and speech difficulties;
- headaches, which can include migraine-like symptoms;

- gastrointestinal or IBS-type symptoms;
- anxiety and depression;
- other symptoms, such as feeling too hot or cold, restless legs, tingling, numbness, prickling, or burning sensations in the hands and feet; tinnitus; and painful periods for women.

You may notice that many of these symptoms are common across the conditions in this book. This is indeed true and is yet another aspect of misunderstood illnesses that make it very challenging for doctors to diagnose. In fact, a diagnosis may be based more on the doctor's speciality than on the symptoms.

To rule out other conditions with similar symptoms to those of FMS, such as CFS/ME (see p. 18), rheumatoid arthritis and multiple sclerosis, blood tests, X-rays and physical examination should be carried out. Once all other conditions have been ruled out, two criteria must be met for a diagnosis of FMS to be confirmed:

- widespread pain must have been present for more than three months on both the left and right sides of the body, both above and below the waist;
- pain must be located in at least 11 of the 18 'tender points' when they are pressed (see Figure 1).

These tender points are the places on the body that are most likely to exhibit pain and where the pain is often at its worst – for example, the neck, inside the shoulder blades and inside the elbows. The symptoms of FMS are often treated with painkillers and other drugs, although physiotherapy and alternative techniques such as acupuncture are sometimes used to alleviate discomfort (see Chapter 6).

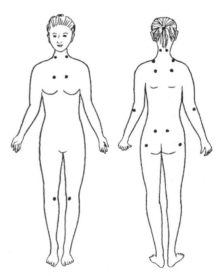

Figure 1 Fibromyalgia syndrome tender points

Chronic fatigue syndrome/ myalgic encephalomyelitis (CFS/ME)

CFS/ME is a much less common condition, affecting up to 3 per cent of the population. As can be gleaned from its name, the primary characteristic is severe fatigue. However, it is misleading to think that CFS/ME causes only fatigue; there are many other symptoms that define this illness. Like all these conditions, it is more common in women than men and appears more likely to develop between the ages of 20 and 40, although children and older people can also be affected. To be diagnosed with CFS/ME all other disorders that could account for the symptoms must be ruled out, and symptoms must have been present for at least six months. Four of the following eight symptoms also need to be present:

- cognitive impairment – problems with memory or concentration
- sore throat
- tender lymph nodes under the arms or on the side of the neck
- muscle pain
- multi-joint pain
- headaches (of a new type, pattern or severity at onset)
- unrefreshing sleep
- post-exertion malaise (extreme tiredness after activity, which lasts more than 24 hours).

Although CFS/ME is not a psychological disorder, psychosocial treatments to help people cope with the illness are recommended by the National Institute of Health and Care Excellence (NICE) in the UK. These include cognitive behavioural therapy (CBT) and graded exercise therapy (GET). However, there are other options (see Chapters 6 and 7). This is a somewhat controversial area, as many people with CFS/ME feel frustrated when psychological techniques are offered, but it must be kept in mind that, at present, we still do not know the cause of the condition and it is therefore very hard to develop effective treatments. Other management strategies include pacing, sleep hygiene, and self-help and self-support (see Chapter 6).

Less common invisible illnesses

Ménière's disease

Ménière's disease is another invisible illness, but it differs from the other conditions in that we know a bit more about the mechanisms associated with it, although like IBS, migraine, FMS and CFS/ME, its exact cause is unknown. In Ménière's disease, the endolymph (the fluid contained in the inner ear) is disturbed. Normally the endolymph has a constant volume and a balance of minerals and electrolytes, and it bathes the sensory cells of the inner ear, allowing for regular function. Some people develop hydrops (swelling), which alters the delicate balance of the endolymph. However, there are no vestibular or auditory tests that can diagnose what is termed as endolymphatic hydrops in Ménière's disease, and hence this illness shares the lack of objective medical tests with the conditions discussed here. It is not known what causes these changes, although some researchers and scientists think they could be due to infection, allergies or metabolic alterations.

Ménière's disease is defined by four main symptoms. Vertigo (a feeling that the external surroundings are spinning around, vertically or horizontally) must be present for a positive diagnosis and, in addition, at least one of the following must also be present:

* hearing loss (usually fluctuating)
* tinnitus (a sensation of noises and ringing in the ears)
* aural fullness (a feeling of pressure or fullness, usually just in one ear).

Although pharmacological treatments may reduce acute vertigo spells and dizziness, symptoms rarely disappear entirely. Ménière's disease is a rare condition, only affecting about 0.2 per cent of people in Western societies, although almost 2 per cent of Americans report the symptoms associated with Ménière's disease, so it might be under-diagnosed.

Mal de débarquement syndrome (MdDS)

MdDS is an even less common disorder. It is a neurological condition that affects some people after being on transport, usually a boat or a ship, for a long time. Unfortunately, people who go on to have MdDS do not readily adapt once they disembark, and consequently life becomes very difficult indeed, because the vast majority of the time (or all the time) they feel unsteady, dizzy and have bobbing and rocking sensations – they feel as if they were still on a ship or other transport. MdDS can be triggered by air or car travel as well, or even funfair rides and motion-based games. The symptoms can last for months or even years. For every nine women who have MdDS, there is one man.

Since MdDS is so rare, finding a doctor who will refer you to a neurologist, and obtaining a diagnosis, can be very difficult. As there is no effective treatment for MdDS, people with it have to manage their condition as best they can. Luckily there are websites run by people with MdDS. Since giddiness and dizziness are symptoms of this disorder, healthy people who hear about this disorder naturally think of 'problems in the inner ear', but this is not the case. It is not known why people fail to adapt to being on land again.

It might be thought that Ménière's disease is similar to MdDS, but there are more differences than similarities. Vertigo, the main symptom of Ménière's disease, is not present in people with MdDS, medications that are effective in Ménière's disease are not effective in MdDS, and people with Ménière's disease do not feel a constant sense of bobbing and rocking.

What do these conditions have in common?

Origin

All the illnesses in this book are of unknown origin – doctors and scientists do not know their exact causes. Most researchers accept that there may be a genetic component and that you may be more likely to develop the condition if a member of your family has it. However, this appears to be just a small piece of the puzzle and in all the invisible illnesses there are normally triggering factors. This is clearest in MdDS, as the symptoms usually start after travelling. When people first started researching CFS/ME, it appeared that viral infections were the cause (such as the virus that causes glandular fever, Epstein–Barr virus (EBV)). However, it was later discovered that many people without CFS/ME also had antibodies to EBV, and hence the answer was not quite so simple.

Symptoms

A great many of the symptoms of these disorders are the same. Fatigue is very common, though it may not be one of the diagnostic symptoms that a GP will look for in migraine or Ménière's disease. However, sometimes a symptom such as fatigue may be the very distinguishing factor for a diagnosis (see Chapter 5); people with IBS can experience significant fatigue, and those with CFS/ME will often have IBS-like symptoms, so it is the *nature* of the fatigue that may lead to one diagnosis rather than another. If the fatigue is much worse after activity (post-exertional fatigue) and it takes a very long time to recover, then a diagnosis of CFS/ME could be more likely, even if symptoms such as constipation or diarrhoea are present. Likewise, some people who have migraines but who are not diagnosed with Ménière's disease have vertigo before, during or after an attack. This is one of the reasons that it may take a long time to get a diagnosis – it can be very difficult for doctors to decide the best diagnosis when there are no objective tests (see Chapter 6).

Diagnosis

All these invisible illnesses are diagnosed by the exclusion of other conditions that could account for the symptoms. In Ménière's disease and MdDS, for instance, all other vestibular disorders such as acoustic neuroma (a benign, slow-growing tumour that develops from the balance and hearing nerves supplying the inner ear), vestibular neuritis and labyrinthitis (both caused by an infection that inflames the inner ear) are first ruled out. This can obviously take time and it may be difficult to find a specialist who can help.

Even once a diagnosis is made, the situation can still be extremely confusing for both doctors and patients. One research study found that in specialist clinics, 70 per cent of people with FMS also fulfilled the diagnostic criteria for CFS/ME. Another study illustrated that nearly 66 per cent of participants with the primary complaint of FMS reported fatigue as a major symptom and that 20 per cent met diagnostic criteria for CFS/ME. Yet another study found that 15 per cent of a community-based sample of people diagnosed with CFS/ME met the criteria for FMS. Conversely, almost a quarter of people diagnosed with FMS were also diagnosed with CFS/ME. These findings are perhaps unsurprising, because nearly 80 per cent of people with FMS experience fatigue as one of their core symptoms, and pain is often a debilitating symptom in CFS/ME. It may be the case that a particular diagnosis is more reliant on the specialism of the doctor than the symptoms *per se* – a rheumatologist could be more likely to diagnose FMS, whereas an immunologist or a virologist might diagnose CFS/ME. A neurologist could label a set of symptoms as 'migraine', although an ear, nose and throat (ENT) specialist might say the condition is Ménière's disease. This is why it can be very important for you, the patient, to disentangle the myriad of symptoms to help your doctor come to the best conclusion (see Chapter 6).

Should these illnesses be lumped together?

Because there are so many similarities within these 'functional' syndromes (see Chapter 1: a condition is labelled as functional if the problem seems to be a fault in the way the body system works, rather than the symptoms being due to an actual disease process), some theorists have proposed that all of these illnesses should be lumped together under the umbrella of 'functional somatic syndrome'. Indeed, with the overlap in diagnoses, the meaningfulness of separating these conditions into distinct illnesses has been questioned. One study tried to tackle this question by looking at the history leading up to a diagnosis of CFS/ME as opposed to IBS to see if important differences could be identified. In 2006, researchers observed 592 people who had an acute attack of gastroenteritis caused by *Campylobacter* bacteria and 243 people who had glandular fever (which is caused by EBV) for six months. The research found that people who had gastroenteritis were significantly more likely to go on to develop IBS than CFS/ME. The researchers also found that people who had had glandular fever were more likely to become chronically ill with CFS/ME than IBS. This research showed that there are important differences between IBS and CFS/ME, namely the 'precipitating' factors. It is important to point out that not everyone who had these infections developed either IBS or CFS/ME (only 56 people with gastroenteritis were diagnosed with IBS six months afterwards, and only 16 of those with glandular fever were diagnosed with CFS/ME in the same time period), which shows that these conditions are not an inevitable consequence of having these infections.

How do acute triggers turn into long-term conditions?

Although not every case of every invisible condition will have a trigger factor, many do. These can be infections as mentioned above, other physical trauma like a road traffic accident or surgery or even environmental toxins such as high levels of pesticides. The trauma may not necessarily be physical; it can also be emotional or psychological, such as abuse as a child, the loss of a loved one, being made redundant or simply having an overwhelmingly busy life. There is now a greater appreciation of how emotional triggers actually produce the same physiological changes within the body as physical triggers.

Therefore, there are a range and variety of triggering events, but this still does not explain how an acute event can start the process of long-term ill health. In some conditions (CFS/ME, IBS and FMS), personality has been viewed as a perpetuating or maintaining factor – for instance, being very perfectionistic, having high standards and tending to be hard on oneself. This may be because people with these types of personalities do not allow their bodies enough time to recover from the trigger before returning to their work and roles. An interesting study that looked at how 'driven' people were before they became ill with either IBS or CFS/ME found that people who were more hard-driving (that is, who pushed themselves very hard to achieve) developed these conditions.

The extent to which we think we can control our lives and illness has also been shown to be a maintaining factor in these conditions, with people who feel they have some control over the illness generally doing better (see Chapter 6).

Finally, depression (see Chapter 4) can also be an important aspect of long-term conditions, although it doesn't necessarily follow that people who are depressed will be worse off. Some researchers have suggested that there is an interaction between fatigue and depression, in that one increases the risk of the other.

In addition to the triggering and perpetuating factors, there may also be predisposing aspects that would make it more likely for people to develop these illnesses. There does seem to be a genetic predisposition in these disorders, particularly IBS, migraine and CFS/ME. Another predisposing factor may be low-grade trauma – rather than a harsh event in life or an infection, an environment that lacks warmth and compassion and also constant autoimmune activation in the form of allergies have been linked to some of these conditions. These constant, but not dramatic, attacks on the physiology may make a person more susceptible to developing a long-term condition in the face of additional demands, such as a major life event like a divorce or an acute viral infection.

Why more women than men?

Some invisible illnesses have a clear hormonal link, such as migraine. However, this is just one type of migraine, known as 'pure menstrual migraine', where hormones are the trigger factors. In this specific kind of migraine, attacks tend to occur at the point in the menstrual cycle where oestrogen is at its lowest. It is most common in women in their 40s. But this does not explain why more women than men have migraines and why more women than men are diagnosed with the other conditions in this book.

One theory concerns stress. Stress is believed to be a perpetuating factor as well as a trigger in these conditions. Our bodies are programmed to deal with acutely stressful events by altering our physiology. When a danger is presented, our bodies react in such a way as to increase our chances of survival – our awareness is heightened, our heart rate increases and hormones are released. This aids the 'fight or flight response', a primitive and automatic reaction to a threat. Our hunter–gatherer ancestors would have been confronted with many serious threats to survival in the form of large animals. If such a threat were to present itself, the fight or flight response would allow them to make a very quick decision about whether to stay and fight (perhaps in the process also securing dinner!) or to run. Within this state of physiological and psychological hyper-arousal, there is a boost of speed and strength to give the best possible chance of survival. This is achieved by the activation of the autonomic nervous system and the endocrine system, specifically the hypothalamic–pituitary–adrenal (HPA) axis (see Chapter 4). These processes are extremely intricate, involving a great deal of interactions between our bodily systems and organs.

The HPA axis is the regulatory system that connects the central nervous system with the hormonal system in our bodies. Under times of acute stress, the HPA axis triggers a process that ends with the secretion of cortisol (sometimes known as the stress hormone). Cortisol is vital in the fight or flight response because it mobilizes resources within the body to provide additional energy, which helps to deal with the increased demand in times of acute stress. Additionally, cortisol aids the regulation of the immune system, cardiac system and many other affective (mood) and cognitive processes. Hence, this is the mechanism for the increased heart rate, heightened mental awareness and other phenomena that occur when the hunter comes across a bear!

These are all obviously advantageous processes but sometimes, if a person is exposed to high levels of stress for extended periods, the bodily systems cannot reach homoeostasis, or rather a state of balance. Indeed, people with FMS and CFS/ME have been found to have a disturbance in their HPA axis, and it is generally accepted that heightened stress is involved in many diseases, including cancer and cardiovascular disease.

However, the question still exists as to why this should be more relevant to women than men. Recently, it has been acknowledged that men and women have differing stress responses – whereas men experience 'fight or flight', women react in a 'tend or befriend' manner. This makes sense if we think about our hunter–gatherer ancestors again. The men would have been on the plains catching dinner (of course this is very simplistic, as we know that only 10 per cent of the diet consisted of meat from hunting), while the women would have their own, different, survival threats to contend with. For example, they would need to 'tend' for their children to ensure the survival of the next generation and also 'befriend' others in order to link with social groups to provide protection and to increase resources. These types of care-giving behaviours are dependent on sex-linked hormones. This is a very new area of enquiry in scientific research but it does appear that men and women (on average) do react differently in a *physiological* sense in times of stress. Indeed, a review of the academic literature found that men had higher cortisol responses to stress than women and that this lower response in women may be related to a hypo-reactivity (under-reactivity) of the HPA axis, which is associated with an increased risk of autoimmune diseases, FMS and CFS/ME.

Another aspect of the greater number of women than men with these conditions may be the way in which doctors diagnose a set of apparently vague symptoms. Doctors are more likely to diagnose a woman with CFS/ME or FMS than they are a man. Therefore, a doctor's perception could be important here. Also, men visit their GP less often than women and may have symptoms that are simply unreported. Again, this is unlikely to be the complete answer here but it could well be a part of the picture.

Summary and conclusion

In this chapter we have outlined a number of invisible and often misunderstood illnesses. Theories and evidence regarding how acute infections and trauma can develop into long-term conditions have been discussed. Finally, by looking at the different responses to stress between men and women, we have sought to answer the question as to why more women than men become ill with these disorders. In Chapter 3 we continue this discussion of commonalities in these invisible and misunderstood illnesses by exploring the stigma associated with these illnesses, illness intrusiveness and impact on one's life. In Chapter 4 depression, anxiety and sleep disturbance are discussed, since these are also shared characteristics of invisible illnesses.

3

Living with a chronic illness

A person suffering from a chronic illness is shaken to one's foundations. Their most basic identity with associated roles is challenged. (Delmar et al., 2005, p. 208)

This chapter discusses the challenges posed by adapting to living with a chronic illness, including any feelings of guilt and anxiety you may have and the need to deal with the attitudes of others, which can sometimes be less than supportive. This is especially relevant if you suffer from an illness where you look well, where you haven't any clear diagnosis or where no one really knows much about it. We talk about the possible effects of illness on different aspects of your life, including relationships with your partner, friends and doctor, and we give vignettes from people who have told us about their experiences of living with a chronic illness.

Psychologists have outlined the stages people go through when adapting to terminal illness. However, long-term illnesses are different, as they do not follow a predictable trajectory. Psychologists have shown how people with certain diseases were able to adapt to their illnesses. However, most of these studies focused on medically legitimized illnesses such as cancer or multiple sclerosis. Living with a condition that is contested or not legitimized has its own particular problems. In addition to unpredictability and a feeling of loss of control, you may feel that others don't believe that your symptoms are real or that you are somehow to blame. When there are no obvious medical reasons for your condition, people around you sometimes give you their 'expert' opinion – it's stress (for most conditions) or something you've eaten (for IBS) or it's a problem in the inner ear (for MdDS). In relation to misunderstood illnesses, research shows that, at first, people feel distressed and anxious, but that in order to cope with it, they – that is, you – have to incorporate it into their life, so that the illness becomes ordinary: you have to learn to manage it.

When you first have a chronic illness that is misunderstood and not legitimized, you feel out of control and robbed of a life you thought you would have, and your identity as the person you thought you were seems fragile. Of course, mixed in with these feelings is the expectation that there will be a medical reason for your symptoms, and that the doctors will find out what causes your symptoms, and then you will get effective treatment and get better. Your friends – and you – might feel optimistic, but as the days turn into weeks and the weeks into months, some friends and family members may become impatient for you to get better and wonder whether there is something you are or are not doing that is hampering your progress. You might worry about this too. Why did I get this illness? Is it something I did? Am I going mad? There will be times when symptoms recede and times when they become worse, apparently at random.

The first hurdle: diagnosis

People with misunderstood illnesses face significant challenges, the first of which is getting the correct diagnosis. We have talked before about the importance of medical legitimization, but to have friends and family who validate and legitimize your illness is also important. Research in 2007 showed that some people with CFS/ME experienced significant delay in getting a diagnosis, and that their doctors were sceptical about them and disrespectful, making a diagnosis of depression or affective disorder (mood disorder) without considering other diagnoses. Worse, though, was when family members doubted, because the person who was ill viewed the doubt and delegitimization as personal rejection, and felt hurt by it. It has been found that FMS has severe negative physical, mental and social impacts that at times can become intrusive and overwhelming. As in the other conditions, the diagnosis of FMS is contested, and sometimes medical people don't really think there's much wrong with you because there is no 'medical evidence'. So you may feel you might have to fight for a diagnosis, and you worry whether people will believe you.

People with FMS have severe pain, which of course is invisible to others. Friends and partners often see that the person with the illness looks well and that the symptoms of the illness are variable. These factors lead them to be sceptical about the illness, which makes it more likely that you will think twice about telling other people about your disorder. IBS is also a misunderstood illness, as there is still no agreement on the exact cause(s) of IBS, and the symptoms are variable and, in the main, invisible. As healthy people often suffer from indigestion, stomach pain, diarrhoea and constipation at some time in their lives, they often believe they know what IBS feels like. However, having these symptoms occasionally does not relate to the misery felt if you have IBS.

I was told there was nothing wrong with me. This annoyed me a lot, as there obviously *was* something not right. Doctors shouldn't tell people there's nothing wrong – I felt as if I was wasting my doctor's time when there were real patients for him to deal with. Later I came to the conclusion that he didn't think I was just making it up, that he really meant that they couldn't *find* anything wrong. But at the time I felt really low.

(RR, with IBS)

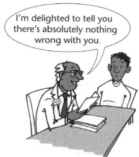

Reproduced by kind permission of Jacky Fleming

There are no biological markers (such as substances that can be measured in the blood, showing that someone is likely to have a certain disease or condition) for IBS, and most medications are ineffective for most people most of the time. Without a clear medical explanation, there is a tendency for others to think that anxiety (or depression) can cause the symptoms. Psychosocial factors do influence the course of IBS, as they do in other conditions. Research shows that anxiety can trigger a worsening of symptoms, and that people feel out of control and embarrassed. Moreover, they don't like to disclose their illness to others. Fatigue, pain, and restrictions in activities and foods affect all aspects of life. All misunderstood illnesses have these types of problems.

Feelings you might have

Guilt

You may feel guilty that you have a chronic illness, that you are adversely affecting the lives of your partner, family, friends and colleagues. You may feel guilty that you arrange to go out for social events or holidays, and have to cancel. You may feel guilty that you have to depend on people. Sometimes people feel guilty because they think that they may have contributed to their illness in some way. These feelings may be ill defined and the person may not *really* believe this, but often people search for something they may have done – or not done – that influenced the course of the illness.

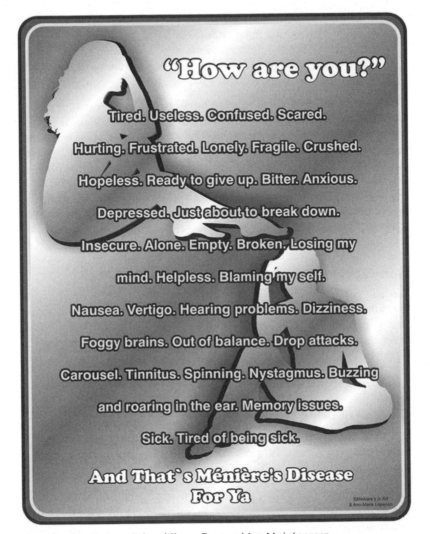

"How are you?"

Tired. Useless. Confused. Scared. Hurting. Frustrated. Lonely. Fragile. Crushed. Hopeless. Ready to give up. Bitter. Anxious. Depressed. Just about to break down. Insecure. Alone. Empty. Broken. Losing my mind. Helpless. Blaming myself. Nausea. Vertigo. Hearing problems. Dizziness. Foggy brains. Out of balance. Drop attacks. Carousel. Tinnitus. Spinning. Nystagmus. Buzzing and roaring in the ear. Memory issues. Sick. Tired of being sick.

And That's Ménière's Disease For Ya

Reproduced by kind permission of Shayne Town and Ann-Marie Loponen.

However, you didn't choose to have this illness. If you were totally healthy, wouldn't you help loved ones if they had a similar illness?

Embarrassment

It was not easy managing my IBS around other people, however. I was initially very worried about the risks posed by eating. My solution was to avoid being around my friends for long periods of time when eventually it would be necessary to eat. I would eat at home whenever I could, where there was the guarantee of privacy and an infinite supply of tissues to spit out the fluid in my mouth. I envisioned these extreme measures helped reduce my having to cover up the embarrassing symptoms, though there were social consequences.   (SB, with IBS)

Chronic illness does have some embarrassing symptoms. It's hard being dependent on people, or having to rush to the toilet, or having to have help in getting to the toilet or having a shower. Bowel incontinence is also embarrassing. It's natural to be embarrassed but the embarrassment itself is probably the least of your problems! Doctors have seen it all, and friends and family will get used to it and will gradually forget embarrassing episodes that you yourself will probably remember for a very long time. Most people have said or done embarrassing things in their lives; they understand.

Worry about letting people down

You will worry too about the possibility of letting people down when you are not well enough to go out to social occasions, or you worry that you can't look after your family properly or go to work. Many people spend time worrying about all sorts of things which might – or might not – happen. Obviously these worries will come into your mind every so often, but rumination will worsen your psychological health. This is a time to put yourself first!

A feeling of being stigmatized

You may feel stigmatized and that people are treating you differently because of your illness. People with chronic illness may feel a sense of shame about their illness. You may feel that others will judge you and have negative attitudes towards you.

It's difficult coping with a chronic condition, and most people don't like to draw attention to themselves and their illness. Many prefer not to tell others of the symptoms. It's hard for people to understand and support you if you don't tell them about your illness, but of course that itself might lead them to treat you differently.

It is deeply upsetting being fobbed off, mocked, and generally dismissed – you tell people you are ill, but they make their own minds up. 'You're just being lazy,' 'You need to join a tennis club,' 'You're just depressed.' None of these is helpful! Of everyone, the medical 'professionals' have been the worst. Infuriatingly so!   (CR, with CFS/ME)

Stigma is usually related to shame. For example, people with certain illnesses might need to get to the toilet quickly. Talk of bowel habits is still quite unacceptable in Western society, and so people with this symptom may feel that others laugh at them behind their back. Contested illnesses such as CFS/ME, IBS and FMS tend to attract more stigma than cancer, for instance. Researchers have stated that patients with illnesses such as CFS/ME often feel that their experience of being physically ill is not validated and that the higher levels of stigma in this group is likely to be a consequence of the ambiguity regarding the cause of the condition.

One way to reduce the stigma attached to illnesses is to talk about them, giving others information about the illness and its effects. Disclosing personal information about yourself can be very difficult. However, doing so is likely to reduce the stigma you feel and to raise the profile of your illness, thereby indirectly helping everyone with the illness. Concealing symptoms has been found to relate to higher levels of depression.

A feeling that the illness affects every part of your life – illness intrusiveness

Illness intrusiveness is a concept devised by Professor Gerald Devins, a psychologist in Canada. He constructed a 13-item questionnaire that covers the extent to which an illness intrudes into your life. The aspects are:

1 health
2 diet
3 work
4 active recreation (such as sports)
5 passive recreation (such as reading)
6 financial situation
7 relationship with partner
8 sex life
9 family relations
10 other social relations
11 self-expression and self-improvement
12 religious expression
13 community and civic involvement.

People rate each statement on how intrusive the illness is into each particular domain (1 = not at all intrusive through to 7 = highly intrusive). Scores can then be added to give a total illness intrusiveness score.

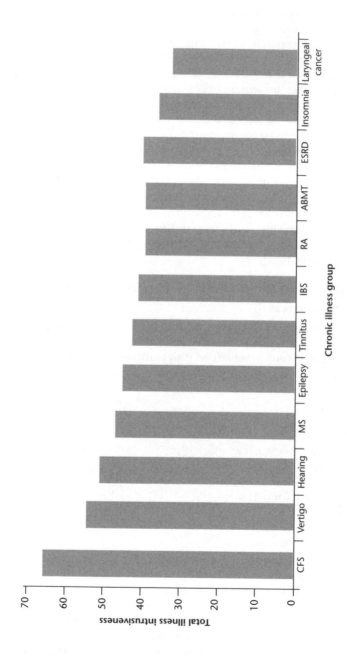

Figure 2 Illness intrusiveness by condition

Any chronic illness intrudes into your life. IBS, for instance, intrudes mostly into relationships with partners and friends and into travel. Travel is especially difficult because of the need to access toilet facilities. CFS/ME intrudes primarily into work and finance (many people with CFS/ME have to give up work or reduce hours) and also into important relationships. The extent to which an illness interferes with one's life depends on various factors – the age of the person and the type of illness, for instance. However, the higher the illness intrusiveness, the more likely it is that depression will result.

Total illness intrusiveness scores are available for hundreds of different conditions. Figure 2 shows just a few of them.

You can see that CFS/ME and two symptoms of Ménière's disease (vertigo and hearing problems) are more intrusive than illnesses such as multiple sclerosis and rheumatoid arthritis and even laryngeal (throat) cancer.

How illness intrusiveness may affect you

People with CFS/ME find that their illness is most intrusive in active recreation, health, work and finance, which is similar to people with migraine (health, work, active recreation) and IBS (diet, health, active recreation and self-expression). As you would expect, the unpredictability of an illness, in terms of causes, diagnosis, treatment, symptom severity and frequency, make illness intrusiveness worse. And when the illness is highly intrusive, then quality of life is reduced.

This probably comes as no surprise to you. However, what might be surprising is that other factors, such as feeling stigmatized, affects the way in which illness intrusiveness reduces your quality of life. So if two people have identical scores on illness intrusiveness, then the one who feels highly stigmatized will have a lower quality of life than the one who doesn't feel so much stigma. This means that you might be able to reduce the stigma you feel by coming out about your illness, finding out lots of information about the illness and telling others, going to self-help groups and undergoing counselling. Reducing the stigma should lead to lower illness intrusiveness and a better quality of life. One study found that group psychotherapy reduced the intrusiveness of systemic lupus erythematosus and helped patients adapt to the illness. We do not know of any other studies which have been carried out in this area.

Other effects of illness on life

Employment

A proportion of working people with chronic illness either resign or are dismissed from their jobs. People with CFS/ME and MdDS are more likely than people with migraine or IBS to have this problem.

Research into the effects of MdDS are rare, but in one of only two studies we found, the researchers noted that 54 per cent reported a reduction in income due to MdDS and they also found that 10 per cent had been dismissed. In our own study of MdDS, we found that a number of people with MdDS changed jobs, or took a reduction in hours, to help them to cope more easily.

For CFS/ME, different studies estimate that between 35 and 69 per cent of people are unemployed, and rates of job loss are estimated to be 26–89 per cent. Those who were still in work had significant work-related disability.

A study on people with FMS showed that the percentage of people in work fell from 60 per cent to 49 per cent in the first three months of having FMS. Twelve months later, the employment rate had fallen to 41 per cent.

A reduction in employment applies to all long-term conditions. Misunderstood illnesses have economic costs for the country as well. When there are no effective treatments for these conditions, when they are not taken seriously and when health professionals cannot help you to cope effectively, then it is likely that you will need multiple visits to the GP or hospital, will need regular medications, will need to take periods of sick leave from employment and may need state benefits. When the illness affects the financial situation, then family relationships may become strained.

Relationships with others

Health professionals

In 2009 Professor Elke Van Hoof in Belgium looked at how 177 patients with CFS/ME felt about their experiences with their GP. According to the patients, only 35 per cent of the GPs showed experience in CFS/ME, and only 23 per cent had sufficient knowledge to treat the condition. Professor Van Hoof said that the controversy surrounding CFS/ME made medical encounters difficult, and that the patients seemed dissatisfied with their interactions with their GP. GPs know even less about MdDS – it has been found that a large number of health-care visits are required before a diagnosis is obtained. The diagnosis of Ménière's disease is also difficult, and quite often a diagnosis of Ménière's disease is given to people who complain of dizziness before they are referred to a specialist such as an ENT surgeon or a neurologist. The diagnosis of Ménière's disease often takes time because there are symptoms that could be a result of other disorders, and these need to be ruled out.

In an early study of people with IBS by our team, we found that many people did not have good relationships with their doctors and felt let down by them. We also found that when people with IBS had the same view as their doctors (about the possible causes of their IBS), they had better interactions than when the doctors had one view (such as stress) and their patients had a totally different view (such as a medical cause). A more recent study (2011) of people with IBS found that interactions were still difficult. In fact, in this study the majority of patients viewed the relationships negatively. They didn't feel they were being listened to properly or that they had received empathy. It is somewhat depressing that not much seems to have changed, even though we now know more about IBS than we did years ago!

Partner and family

Your relationship with your partner naturally changes when you are ill. Research shows that the more fluctuations or changes in CFS/ME symptoms, the more adaptation is required by the couple. One study in the UK found that half of 389 people with migraine said that because of their migraine they were more likely to argue with their partner, children and work colleagues.

Some families are able to cope with problems due to illness, but others find it overwhelming. Strains in partner and family relationships adversely affect health. Studies have shown that marital conflict affects the HPA axis and compromises the immune system. These mechanisms may be the cause of worsening symptoms in chronic illness. After diagnosis people often complain that they are left on their own to deal with their chronic illness, and sometimes they have no idea which way to turn. One article about FMS states that family therapists should focus on pain-coping techniques, dealing with depression, addressing partnership issues and fostering emotional support, and that they should set up a recovery programme. This could be something you could talk to your health practitioner about!

Research into partners of people with chronic illness show that life can change immensely for the partner, who previously might have had interests and hobbies that could be pursued easily. Once a family member has a chronic illness, the partner might have to take on the bulk of the housework and cooking, despite having to go to work. Instead of simply being able to go out, complex arrangements might have to be made in advance. For instance, researchers in Sweden found that the whole family is affected when the woman in the family has FMS. Relationships changed between the partners, as the other had to take on greater responsibility and participation in childcare and upbringing.

> When Katrina first became ill, we thought it was a flu-like illness and she would get over it soon, but as she gradually got worse it was obviously something more serious. Eventually she was spending all day and night in bed unable to do anything. This, to put it mildly, was inconvenient for me! Not only did I have to do a full day's work and frequently get shopping on the way home, I had to cope with cooking – which is not my strong point – and do all the housework and look after the cats. While I was doing this I felt guilty that I wasn't sitting with Katrina as she had been alone all day. We did sit together to eat our dinner off trays (she was in bed) so at least we were together then. I usually managed to read children's stories to her last thing at night (she couldn't cope with more advanced books!), which she enjoyed, especially when I made all different voices, as you do when reading to young children. Also, as with reading bedtime stories to young children it was very difficult for me to stay awake! Sometimes I had to drive home in my lunch hour to get some food and drink for Katrina and eat mine very quickly before driving back to work. The worst was not knowing how long this illness would last as it seemed unlike a normal illness – it just went on and on, and sometimes I was just totally exhausted. The most difficult thing for me was trying to cope with her being depressed (which she wasn't before). It was difficult to empathize fully with someone who needed so much care. Sometimes I felt resentful, especially when we didn't know how long this was going to go on for. (MJ, whose partner has ME)

In addition to the increased burden of daily chores and activities, the stress of taking care of another person can have an impact on carers' immune function. In the field of psychoneuroimmunology, which looks at the relationship between mentalistic or psychological processes and the immune system, researchers Kiecolt-Glaser, McGuire and colleagues have found that people who care for their spouses heal less quickly than non-carers. Also, when given a vaccination for the influenza virus, carers were less likely to have the appropriate immune response to the vaccine than non-carers. Therefore, it is not just the everyday difficulties that caregivers face – there is a real issue with the impact on carers' health. This is why it is important that people who care for others should develop support networks and ask for help; not only when it's needed, but on a regular basis to prevent illness.

Effects on recreation

When you have a chronic illness, your limited energy needs to be spent doing the things that are absolutely necessary. People who go to work may find they haven't got the energy to take exercise or go out socially. So hobbies and interests tend to be the first things to go. Active recreation (such as sports) may be impossible. Passive recreation (such as reading, listening to music) is not affected so much. However, for people with Ménière's disease, passive recreation *is* affected – hearing problems and tinnitus can obviously intrude into previously valued hobbies and interests. People with migraine can't do as many household chores as previously, and they have to cancel family, social and leisure activities – and a third of them avoid making plans because they are worried about having to cancel them. All the disadvantages of making social appointments and finding that you have to cancel them, or of having to make complex plans to ensure you can actually get to your appointments, mean that sometimes it is just easier to stay at home. However, if you do this too much, your world narrows, and depression might set in. Somehow, you've got to get yourself to a place where you can pull yourself out of the quagmire.

Summary and conclusion

This chapter has discussed the psychosocial consequences of having a chronic illness. We have shown that adapting to a chronic illness is very difficult indeed, particularly when you have an illness that is misunderstood. We have shown that all such illnesses are intrusive, some more than others, and that the feelings of guilt, anxiety and depression that you may feel when you have a chronic illness are normal. Although we haven't got all the answers, we hope that the material in the next chapters will enable you to take back some control over your illness.

4

Stress, depression, anxiety, fatigue and sleep disturbance

> For many individuals with a chronic illness, fatigue is one of their most pervasive and debilitating symptoms.
>
> (Parker White and White, 2011)

Understanding the fight or flight response and the way in which stress affects both your mind and your body, as well as ways in which you might respond to chronic and acute stress, is key to understanding the material in the chapters that follow. Immunity and inflammation are also related to chronic illness. This chapter looks at the ways in which stress, depression, anxiety, fatigue and sleep disturbance are related to one another in all the conditions covered in this book.

Although some people think that psychological states can actually cause an illness, in our opinion these are more likely to be a consequence of living with an intrusive illness that shows no signs of going away any time soon, and that is misunderstood or thought to be trivial by other people. We know that illness can cause you to feel depressed, anxious and worried, and we know that these psychological states can aggravate your illness. There seems to be no way in which we can be certain that depression, say, is a cause, rather than a consequence, of illness. Studies show that diseases such as cancer, AIDS and cardiovascular disease can be *accelerated* by depressed mood (so that the illnesses get worse more quickly than would otherwise be the case). Depression, stress, anxiety, often accompanied by fatigue and sleep disturbances, are common in people with chronic illness. Anxiety and stress can affect long-term illness, and living with a chronic illness can increase anxiety and stress, so we will now discuss some of the physiological processes involved. First of all, think about the nervous system.

The nervous system

The nervous system consists of the central nervous system and the peripheral nervous system, which is then sub-divided further (see Figure 3).

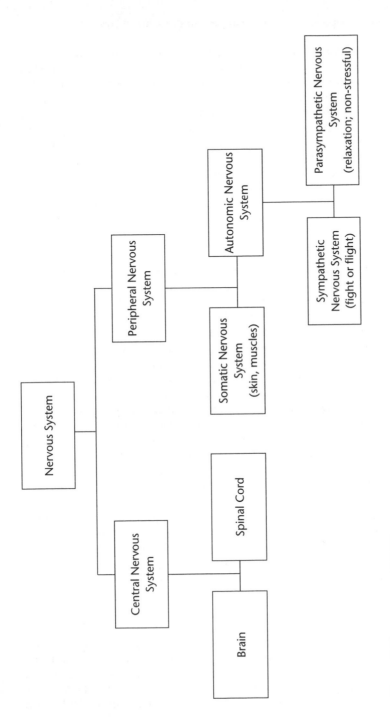

Figure 3 The nervous system

The autonomic nervous system consists of the sympathetic and para-sympathetic systems. The sympathetic nervous system is activated in emergency or stressful situations – your heart rate increases, you begin to perspire and blood is diverted from the gastrointestinal system to the muscles. This is the system that is activated in the fight or flight response. The parasympathetic part of the autonomic nervous system promotes relaxation, and it functions under normal, non-stressful conditions. This system slows the heart rate. These two systems are opposed to each other. This is important because you can reduce stress by meditation. While you're meditating, your parasympathetic nervous system will be activated, so it is not then possible for your sympathetic nervous system to be activated.

Fight or flight response

Imagine you have a near-miss when you are driving or that you have just had a shock. Immediately the sympathetic part of the autonomic nervous system prepares for this emergency. The central nervous system (CNS) is alert and aroused, your pulse rate rises, the adrenal glands release the hormones adrenaline and noradrenaline in response to the stress, and your whole body is geared up to deal with the threat or emergency.

In the examples of the near-miss in a car or a major shock, you normally have no need to run away or fight anyone, but your body nevertheless reacts with the same physiological changes that you might feel if a wild animal was chasing you! This immediate response is followed by slower activation of the HPA axis. The hypothalamus is a part of the brain that communicates with the nervous and endocrine systems, through the pituitary and adrenal glands. If the acute stress of a near-miss (or other type of stress) is over in seconds, and you calmly drive on, the HPA system might not even kick in. However, if the stress continues, the HPA system will be activated, and various hormones will be released into the blood stream – stress hormones such as adrenaline and cortisol, which increases blood sugar levels and metabolic rate. When the stress is over, the HPA system is able to reset itself so that it is back to normal. That is, the HPA system is able to regulate itself. The body is well prepared for such acute, short-term stresses.

However, with longer periods of stress the HPA may be less able to regulate itself, and in this case may stay on 'high-activation' mode. Research shows that such a change in the activity of the HPA system (dysregulation) leads to a suppression of the immune system, and if stress continues, your body can be overwhelmed and you could succumb to illness or burn-out. The HPA system also gives rise to an inflammatory response in the body. Dysregulation of the HPA axis is associated with some long-term conditions, including CFS/ME, and also with emotional states such as depression, but this is not to say that CFS/ME and depression are one and the same.

You may wonder why inflammation occurs, given that it doesn't seem a good thing for you. However, inflammation is a defence mechanism. The inflammatory response inactivates or eliminates viruses and bacteria. For short time-periods, there is no problem, but when you have chronic illness, you may have low-grade, long-term inflammation. Many diseases and disorders have chronic inflammation, including IBD, asthma, possibly IBS and others.

Chronic stress

Chronic stress is more harmful than acute stress. Maybe you work in a stressful environment – perhaps you are very overworked and have an unsympathetic line manager as well as trying to cope with an unpredictable and misunderstood illness. We are sure you can think of many scenarios which apply to your own life! In that case the sympathetic nervous system will be in a state of alert, ready for fight or flight situations. Stress affects both the sympathetic nervous system and the HPA axis. With chronic stress, the dysregulation of the HPA system may cause you to have too much or too little cortisol, and abnormal cortisol levels have been associated with fatigue and muscle pain.

So you can see that stress has wide-ranging effects on the brain and body.

Some researchers believe that persistent dysregulation of the stress system might be an important mechanism in both CFS/ME and FMS. They suggest the sympathetic nervous system might be in a persistent 'overdrive' together with an 'underdrive' (or hyporeactivity) of the HPA axis. This leads to a low-grade immune activation, which contributes to fatigue and pain.

It is important to realize that these descriptions of the nervous system and the HPA axis are very much simplified. There are many papers and books that contain detailed information about the HPA axis and its role in illness. But we hope we have given you enough information to show you that chronic stress (or perhaps repeated acute stresses) adversely affect your brain and body, and we hope that later you will be convinced, as we are, that you can, to some extent, counteract the negative effects of stress.

Chronic illness and stress

Once you have a chronic illness, you will have additional stresses – having to explain the illness to others, feeling you can't do things as you used to, feeling guilty that your partner has to put up with you and your illness and so on. Additional stresses can aggravate the situation. There is much research that shows that stress can worsen various illnesses or diseases. For instance, it can alter the course of multiple sclerosis. Perhaps medically unexplained long-term conditions, such as the ones we cover in this book, have more than psychosocial factors (stigma, illness intrusiveness, depression) in common – that is, they also have physiological problems such as HPA dysregulation in common.

Depression

Stress is associated with depression, and depression itself also has physiological consequences. Natural killer cells are white blood cells that are part of the immune system. They can kill cells such as tumour cells. It is very important for natural killer cells to function as they should. As in the case of chronic stress, in depression natural killer cells activity reduces, inflammation occurs and the HPA system remains activated for longer than necessary. Stress inhibits natural killer cells' activity, and it has been shown to worsen autoimmune diseases. One research team discussed depression in relation to inflammation. They looked at 176 studies of inflammatory markers (certain substances in the blood) and stress and depression. The researchers confirmed a significant overall association between depression and a reduction in the function of T cells (which can destroy or deactivate viruses and bacteria). There was also an increase in the circulation of inflammatory substances. Depression can make any illness worse. For example, it can increase the likelihood of a heart attack in people with heart disease. It is thought that substances produced by the brain (called brain proinflammatory cytokines) are involved in depression.

Brain proinflammatory cytokines cause many of the symptoms that you have when you are ill – for example, they play a positive role in helping the immune system to react to invaders, but they increase inflammation and make you feel lethargic and generally unwell. When you have flu or a similar illness, these effects are likely to make you rest, which helps you to recover.

Depression can not only aggravate your illness but may also be a consequence of your illness. As someone with a particular illness, it's not worth your spending a lot of time worrying about cause and effect in respect of depression, because all that matters is that you deal with it. Don't ignore depression. It's important to be honest with yourself and to consider carefully whether you are just sad or down or miserable some of the time (as many healthy people are) or whether it's worse than this – so bad that you realize that you are depressed (in the true sense of the word) most of the time. Depression is more than feeling miserable. Some people might feel ashamed that they are depressed, but you are of course not alone – depression is a common problem, especially in people with a long-term illness.

Depression is particularly likely in illnesses with no known cause and no long-lasting effective treatments. When the illness is invisible and misunderstood, the depression is likely to be worse. Our own research has shown that people with vestibular disorders such as Ménière's disease, and also CFS/ME and IBS, have particularly high levels of depression, higher than in some more 'severe' diseases. This is not surprising, since these conditions are invisible ones that are particularly misunderstood.

When people become ill, they search for the causes of their illness. Knowing that your illness is caused by a virus, for instance, means that you have a physical cause for your illness, and you know that viral infections tend to clear up on their own. Generally you will feel certain that, however awful you feel, this will pass. Inflammatory bowel disease is much more serious than IBS. People with inflammatory bowel disease sometimes have to have sections of their bowels removed. However, people with inflammatory bowel disease know that they have an organic disease (which has a medical cause, even if the cause is not fully known). They know that there are some at least partially effective treatments. They know that nobody will suspect them of malingering or in some way of causing their own illness. This is reassuring, even as their symptoms remain and are causing them to feel awful. People with the illnesses covered in this book do not have that reassurance and so life can be very challenging indeed.

Depression and/or anxiety in most long-term illness conditions

Many studies have shown a relationship between migraine and depression. Depression is twice as common in people with migraine as it is in people without migraine. Migraine is also often associated with sleepiness and fatigue. Researchers have found that dysregulation of the HPA system seems to be involved in both migraine and depression, meaning that one process may underlie both disorders. Stress can trigger migraine attacks, as can too much or too little sleep.

Likewise, people with Ménière's disease also show high depression scores. In our own study of 85 people with Ménière's disease, only two people were not depressed; six were moderately depressed and the other 77 were severely depressed.

Depression and anxiety occur frequently in people with FMS. People with FMS are five times more likely to experience depression than healthy people A recent study found that 21 per cent of people with FMS had anxiety, and 46 per cent had both depression and anxiety. Depression and stress have both been found to worsen the symptoms of FMS.

Traditionally, psychiatrists and others in the medical profession have thought that depression can explain the various symptoms involved in CFS/ME and other medically unexplained disorders. Many people are aware of the label 'psychosomatic', meaning that psychological factors such as depression or anxiety can cause bodily (somatic) symptoms. Some health professionals, often psychiatrists, believe that depression causes IBS and CFS/ME. However, as noted above in the discussion of the HPA axis, symptoms might very well have a neuro-psychophysiosomatic explanation – that is, interactions between neurological conditions, psychological factors and physiological and biological factors together explain your symptoms.

For example, you might have a genetic predisposition to a particular illness (it 'runs in the family'). As a result of stress you might become run down and more likely to become infected with a virus. Once infected, you might become even more stressed because of work or family commitments, and in the initial stages of the illness, you might push yourself even further, to ensure you meet your commitments. Thus physiological and biological factors interact with psychological and social factors. which will affect how long it will take until you recover.

In 2012, researchers Anderson, Maes and Berk concluded that somatic symptoms also have an organic (rather than psychological) explanation. They say, 'Recent data, however, suggest that somatic symptoms additionally have an organic explanation. Consequently, we use the term "physio-somatic" symptoms – in contrast to psycho-somatic symptoms.' Their study reviewed biological and biochemical evidence. They show that both depression and physiosomatic symptoms are significantly associated with inflammation and immune activation. That is, their review led them to believe that an underlying biological explanation could account for symptoms of functional illnesses. This may lend some weight to the view of some theorists who believe that *all* of these illnesses should be lumped together under the umbrella of 'functional somatic syndrome'.

Other researchers have taken blood samples from patients with CFS/ME to measure immunological changes over time. The results confirmed decreases in immune function, which suggested an increased susceptibility to viral and other infections. In addition, the researchers believe that natural killer cell activity might be a useful marker for diagnosing CFS/ME, as one measure of natural killer cell activity was consistently decreased during the year of the study.

Even if depression and CFS/ME (and other functional conditions) have such an explanation, there is still benefit in treating depression. Many people with medically unexplained disorders, believing that their illness has a medical cause, ignore depression, focusing on their symptoms. However, as we have said earlier, depression can make the illness worse. This is something you might wish to consider.

Traditionally IBS has also been associated with depression and anxiety. There has been debate over many years as to whether these psychological factors cause or trigger IBS. Studies have found increased rates of anxiety and depression in people with IBS. Despite that, most people with IBS do not have anxiety or depression. Those who do, however, are more likely to use the health-care system more than those who do not. Quite often people with IBS are anxious about particular symptoms, such as how to deal with diarrhoea or constipation, rather than being anxious in general.

Rumination

Anxiety and depression are made worse by focusing on negative thoughts, and expanding on them – a process called rumination. Healthy people ruminate, of course. If you have a problem or worry, you ruminate by thinking about it, going over it, thinking how you might explain the problem to someone else, even going through whole conversations in your head or constructing emails mentally. Rumination itself is tiring, but stopping ruminating is very hard to do. (See Chapter 7 for help with this.) Rumination and anxiety are related to each other, each making the other worse. In addition, these habits are likely to lead to worse sleep (rumination often happens at night) and to increasing depression. Feeling lonely also contributes to worsening sleep quality and depression. Sometimes the worry that started this chain of events might have been resolved, but if the situation was very stressful, people may play the events back to themselves, sometimes repeatedly, prolonging the event. As we know, doing this has physiosomatic consequences.

There is a theory that, given the same severity of symptoms, some people amplify their symptoms and some de-amplify them. Of course no one would wish to amplify their symptoms, but there are a number of ways this could happen. Psychological factors such as depression, anxiety or stress could amplify symptoms, and immune factors such as proinflammatory cytokines could be involved in amplification.

Sleep

Why is sleep important in illness? Lack of sleep affects the immune system and activates an inflammatory response. Sleep loss is associated with reduction in natural killer cell activity, which is important for the immune system's ability to mount a response to viral infection. There are different types of sleep problems:

- problems with sleep onset so that you toss and turn, but can't seem to fall asleep, and then if you do fall asleep you don't seem to sleep for long before you wake up;
- waking up early in the morning and then not sleeping again.

If you are really unlucky, you might have more than one type of sleep problem! Physical illness can cause disruption to sleep, and of course sleep disruption can make your illness worse.

The circadian rhythm

A circadian rhythm is a roughly 24-hour cycle in the biological and physiological processes of all living things. Brain activities, hormones, eating and sleeping are governed by this cycle. All biological systems are synchronized to this cycle and they co-ordinate our physiology. So, for example, we are biologically programmed to sleep at night and be awake during the day. These cyclical rhythms are governed by 'body-clocks', which tell our bodies when to sleep and when to rise.

Until the mid 1990s it was thought there was only one clock in the body, the suprachiasmatic nucleus (SCN). Now we know that there are dozens of circadian clocks in our body and that the SCN is the co-ordinator of these clocks. They are synchronized by the SCN, using daylight and night-time cycles, metabolic rates, and neurological conditions. Disruption of these clocks leads to psychological, cognitive and physiological problems – for example, the body clocks make it difficult for shift workers to sleep properly. Sleep problems also occur in viral and bacterial illnesses, in CFS/ME, in FMS and in fact in most illnesses.

It's now thought that problems in the circadian rhythms, such as problems with sleep, can actually *cause* illnesses, although we know that illness also causes sleep problems. As we age, the body clocks become less synchronized, which can lead to poor sleep patterns and weakened immunity. However, physical activity has been shown to help to regulate the body clocks.

Fatigue

We have seen above that anxiety, depression, fatigue and sleep all relate to one another. Fatigue is a significant factor in most long-term illnesses, including the ones we discuss in this book. Although people tend to think of fatigue as physical, there are different types of fatigue. When researchers study fatigue, they usually make a distinction between physical fatigue, mental or cognitive fatigue and emotional fatigue. All these types of fatigue affect the quality of life in people with long-term illness.

That people can have mental fatigue as well as physical fatigue is supported by studies that show different patterns of brain activity depending on different types of fatigue. Other studies give participants taxing mental tasks, and later measure their performance on similar tasks and their fatigue levels. Needless to say, their performance becomes worse after the first tasks, and their fatigue becomes greater.

There are general questionnaires that measure fatigue, such as the Multi-dimensional Fatigue Inventory (MFI). However, researchers recognize that although long-term illnesses have fatigue in common, different illness groups may not experience fatigue in exactly the same way. The MFI measures general fatigue, physical fatigue, mental fatigue and emotional fatigue. Also included are measures of reduced activity and reduced motivation, because these factors are associated with fatigue. However, researchers studying specific long-term diseases and conditions have devised illness-specific fatigue questionnaires. For instance, one research team found that there were 12 different types of fatigue in people with rheumatoid arthritis.

CFS/ME researchers Jason and colleagues (2010) found five different states of fatigue experienced by people with CFS/ME:

- post-exertional fatigue, which occurs after physical or mental effort;
- wired fatigue, the 'wired but tired' state referred to in Chapter 3;
- brain fog, or cognitive exhaustion (you forget words, can't add up or can't understand things), often referred to having a muzzy or fuzzy head (after taking part in research studies that require the processing of information, people with CFS/ME and other similar conditions often feel mentally exhausted);
- energy fatigue, in which you feel too tired to do anything, such as getting up to make a cup of tea;
- flu-like fatigue, which is fatigue caused by what appears to be a viral or bacterial illness.

FMS is also associated with significant fatigue, and people with FMS have been found not only to have physical fatigue and muscle weakness but also brain fog. Just like people with CFS/ME, people with FMS have to pace themselves, to decide whether to do one particular activity, such as cleaning, or another, such as going shopping. People who have significant fatigue but who have to go to work often find they have no energy for anything else, including social events. They have to decide on a daily basis how best to use their limited energy resources. Pain on its own is bad enough, but to have fatigue makes everything far worse.

Fatigue is often the main concern for people with chronic illness, rather than other specific symptoms, for fatigue affects all aspects of life and is a bigger predictor of disability than other symptoms. This means that you are likely to have to take sick leave and will feel anxious about whether you will keep your job. This worry and stress can then make the illness worse, so a cyclical pattern can be created through no fault of your own. Ways to break these patterns and to gain the support you need to manage an invisible illness are discussed in Chapter 7.

The other problem with fatigue is that, generally, people can't see how fatigued you really are. When you feel so bad that you can hardly stand, or even hold your head up, it's hard to believe that you might look fine to others. Even talking on the phone might be too difficult for you, but it is hard for other people to understand that. Sometimes friends and family feel personally insulted because you can't cope with visitors or phone conversations. The invisibility of many long-term conditions is a huge problem – when people can't see your symptoms and your fatigue, they find it very difficult to understand. A compounding problem is that some health professionals, including doctors and nurses, seem not to understand fatigue, and, as we have said earlier, medical legitimization is very important in long-term conditions. When the people who should care for you don't accept your fatigue as 'real' and a part of the illness, you feel a lot worse. People with this kind of fatigue have been told they are depressed. They might indeed be depressed, but this does not mean that their depression led to their fatigue. So many long-term conditions are associated with fatigue, including medically explained conditions such as cancer and rheumatoid arthritis, that surely it is more sensible to conclude (even provisionally) that fatigue is a result of the illness, rather than the other way round. Since fatigue is such an important factor in long-term conditions, it is important that health professionals and others recognize the distress it causes.

However, unless there is a known cause of fatigue (such as thyroid problems), it is not possible to cure the problem. Self-management, with support from others, is the way to treat fatigue. As you probably know, sleeping does not necessarily mean you will feel refreshed when you wake up. However, it is important to ensure that you rest, relax and improve the quality of your sleep. (See Chapters 6 and 7 for some tips on how to get good-quality sleep.)

People often think of being fatigued as being very tired, but unless you have experienced the total fatigue characteristic of CFS/ME, and other conditions with significant fatigue, it is impossible to describe it. The fatigue is both mental and physical. In the worst stages of the illness, physical fatigue means being unable to walk even to the next room easily, and once there you need to sit down. Or it may mean not being able to walk without assistance. At other stages it might be possible to make tea or even a snack, but you need to sit down to do it.

It's so very difficult to describe the fatigue and tiredness that I've experienced as it's not just one thing. When I was first ill and bed-bound, my body simply couldn't do anything. I couldn't wash my own hair as the energy it took to keep my arms lifted up was simply too much for me. But my mind was wide awake, which always seemed so odd to me. Like I couldn't really even talk but my brain would be spinning, high or wired almost. The light and noise from the TV was too much for me at the time so I remember staring at the ceiling for hours, days, and in the end it turned out to be two years, and my mind would make-up stories in the patterns. Characters and everything. So while my body seemed to be near-comatose, my mind was active, which was cruel really. Then there is what everyone calls the 'post-exertional fatigue', which I still get now if I overdo it. So like if I go out with friends and try to keep up beyond my limits, I will be exhausted but not really on the day, it will come the next day or even sometimes the day after. I always found that quite strange and again cruel because if the fatigue is delayed by a couple of days I start to think that I haven't got CFS/ME after all!!! If I'm generally run-down, I get the fluey fatigue, which is a real warning sign for me and tells me that I need to be careful and pace myself. I guess lastly is the almighty 'brain-fog' – again it's weird as I often get this after doing too much physically, not mentally, but mostly if I haven't slept well. Basically, it's like my brain is still there, I know it's there but it's behind a wall of fog. I've heard some people say it's like trying to think through treacle, which I think sums it up too. So it's impossible to tell a GP all this in the seven minutes you have, and it's quite annoying when I tell someone I'm tired and they reply, 'Yeah, I'm knackered too,' as it's not really comparable!   (MA, with CFS/ME)

The fatigue can be mental and cognitive (people call this 'brain fog') – you may be unable to think, find the right words or do some tasks like simple addition (important if you try to play scrabble when you have CFS/ME!). You long to go to bed because you feel so fatigued, but when you wake up in the morning, you still feel fatigued. The saying 'wired but tired' refers to the finding that many people with CFS/ME feel over-stimulated or aroused (wired) despite having no energy (tired). This paradox is explained by the over-activity of the nervous system, the effects of which (inflammatory responses and a change in cortisol and cytokines) have, as a side effect, fatigue and also disrupted sleep.

Although the diagnostic criteria for FMS do not include sleep disturbance, disruption of sleep is also associated with fatigue, and an increase in the inflammatory response in people with FMS. One study found that in comparison to healthy people the majority of a sample of 2,580 people with FMS reported that they had difficulty in falling asleep and staying asleep and that they did not feel as though their sleep was refreshing. Sleep disturbances have bi-directional effects on pain and fatigue, such that pain predicts poorer sleep, and sleep difficulties one night predicts increased pain and fatigue the next night. Migraine, too, is associated with sleep problems. People who suffer from migraine often suffer from restless leg syndrome (RLS). This is an annoying condition in which you have an urge to move your legs when you are resting or in bed. Trying not to move your legs makes the urge to move more intense. It's hard to sleep when you have to keep moving your legs. Salas and Kwan (2012, p. S206) say, 'Thus, whether awake or asleep, the RLS patient finds little opportunity for the general restorative behaviors necessary for healthy human functioning, resulting in high rates of comorbidities including depression, anxiety, and hypertension.' RLS obviously makes it difficult for people to fall asleep and stay asleep.

Just as in CFS/ME and FMS, unrefreshing sleep is more common in people with migraine. Sleep problems are known to lead to headaches, and vice versa, but we still don't understand the mechanisms that underlie this relationship. Patients with migraine who sleep less than normal tend to have migraine attacks during the night or on waking and they are often very sleepy during the day. Many people with migraine sleep at irregular times, and this can aggravate symptoms – regular patterns of sleep are key, both for people with migraine and for people with other long-term conditions.

Although Ménière's disease is not associated with fatigue in the way that CFS/ME and FMS are, it has been found that tinnitus may be associated with sleep disturbance, fatigue and depression.

Anecdotal evidence from people with MdDS suggests that stress or lack of sleep aggravates symptoms.

Thus in all these conditions, it is essential to have good-quality sleep; this doesn't refer to quantity but to quality, as we all differ in the amount of sleep we need.

In IBS too, people report sleep problems. Interestingly, a recent study suggested that as people with IBS are hypervigilant, this hyper-arousal might be associated with activation of the HPA axis. Hyper-arousal can lead to sleep disruption. People who are 'wired but tired' might also have sleep disruption because of this problem.

Isn't it interesting that all these different conditions have so much in common?

The stages of sleep

Sleep has five stages, one stage of rapid eye movement (REM) sleep and four stages of non-REM sleep. People start with a light non-REM sleep (stage 1) which becomes deeper (stages 2–4) before they enter REM sleep, which is when most dreams occur. High brain activity occurs during REM sleep. This pattern is repeated throughout the night (see Figure 4, overleaf).

It has been found that stages 3 and 4 are particularly important – studies show that sleep-deprived people are deprived mostly of stages 3 and 4.

Good quality sleep?

Studies show that you need to feel secure to sleep, and this includes feeling secure in key social relationships. Researchers have found that married people who were anxious about their current relationships reported poorer sleep quality, and that women with anxious relationships had a significantly smaller percentage of stages 3 and 4 sleep than others. Even short periods of lost sleep can elevate the stress hormone cortisol.

It is very hard to think about any one of these factors individually, as you can see that there are complex interactions between physio-somatic symptoms, anxiety, stress, depression and sleep, and all these factors affect and are affected by all the other factors. There is also a relationship between pain and sleep. Sleep disruption lowers the pain threshold, so that you are more likely to start feeling pain at a low, rather than a high, intensity; and of course being in pain makes it difficult to sleep.

Improving any one of these will have positive effects on the others. We give you ways to help yourself in Chapter 7.

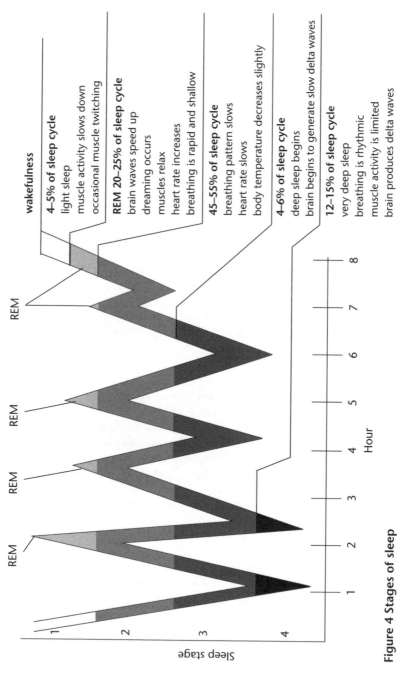

wakefulness

4–5% of sleep cycle
light sleep
muscle activity slows down
occasional muscle twitching

REM 20–25% of sleep cycle
brain waves speed up
dreaming occurs
muscles relax
heart rate increases
breathing is rapid and shallow

45–55% of sleep cycle
breathing pattern slows
heart rate slows
body temperature decreases slightly

4–6% of sleep cycle
deep sleep begins
brain begins to generate slow delta waves

12–15% of sleep cycle
very deep sleep
breathing is rhythmic
muscle activity is limited
brain produces delta waves

REM   REM   REM   REM

Hour

Sleep stage

1   2   3   4   5   6   7   8

1
2
3
4

Figure 4 Stages of sleep

Summary and conclusion

This chapter has shown that the way our bodies react to stress and depression can, through the autonomic nervous system and the HPA axis, worsen our illness. A change in activity of the HPA system may lead to a suppression of the immune system and an inflammatory response in the body. These effects can lead to feeling unwell and fatigued. We have shown that depression, anxiety, worry and rumination can disturb your sleep, increasing your fatigue. This chapter has shown the complex ways in which biological, psychological and social processes interact together to aggravate your illness. In the chapters that follow, we give you ways of helping to cope with the challenges you face when you have a chronic, misunderstood illness.

5

Mind over matter?

By changing our mind, we are changing our brain.
(Paquette et al., 2003)

Anyone who dismisses the power of mind over matter hasn't heard about the amazing effects of the placebo response. This chapter describes studies that have shown that, in medical practice, placebos can be useful because they can help people to get better. It discusses the ways in which both placebos and nocebos can work, and how we can all harness the power of placebos. Placebo and nocebo effects illustrate the way in which mind over matter techniques can be helpful.

Placebo effects

Traditionally, the placebo effect refers to any inactive substance (such as a sugar pill) that has beneficial effects. ('Placebo' in Latin means 'I shall please'.)

You have probably heard that placebo pills have different effects depending on the colour they are. People associate blue pills with calmness, and so in the absence of any information about the way the (placebo) pills work, blue placebo pills produce a tranquillizing effect, whereas orange placebo pills have the opposite effect.

Researchers have studied coffee drinkers. Moderate doses of oral caffeine tablets cause the release of a neurochemical called dopamine. Eight habitual coffee drinkers were scanned after no treatment at all and also after taking placebo tablets. (Participants were told that they had a 50 per cent chance of receiving caffeine but all were given a placebo.) Despite no one receiving caffeine, measurements showed that the participants released the neurochemical dopamine! Although the participants were given inert, inactive pills, the brain released the neurochemical dopamine, just as if they had taken real caffeine pills.

A painkiller such as iboprufen stimulates the body to produce opioids, substances that act against pain. In 1978 researchers found that giving participants a placebo pill (said to be to relieve pain) stimulated the body to produce opioids. So an inactive, inert placebo painkiller is able to stimulate the body to produce opioids. The placebo-activated opioids have also been shown to produce respiratory depression (meaning that you are not able to breathe properly, or hypoventilation), which is a typical side effect of real opioids. So the placebo acts like the real drug and can produce side effects like the real drug!

When drug companies wish to show how effective a drug is, they usually have to show how much more the treatment improves symptoms over and above the improvement attributed to a placebo. In these situations, the placebo is really a nuisance, as it's harder to show real effects of a drug when there are big effects from the placebo. It would be easier to show an effect of the drug if there were no placebo effects. In practice, there are always placebo effects. For instance, take the study we carried out on people with IBS. We gave people a nutritious food supplement to test its effect on six symptoms of IBS. (Constipation was included as a symptom, but the product was not expected to improve this.) Figure 5 shows that symptoms did improve with the supplement more than with the placebo. However, the placebo alone also improved symptoms. The participants weren't told that constipation wasn't expected to improve, but despite that, both the placebo product (which looked identical to the real product) and

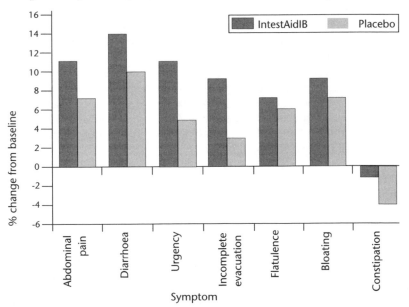

Figure 5 Percentage improvement for both active and placebo treatment

the real product failed to work for constipation! Now that really is weird. Neither the participants nor the researchers (that is, our team) knew whether participants were taking the active tablet or the placebo.

In the case of flatulence, the effect of the active product was very similar to that of the placebo, so that the company that produced the nutritious product would have to conclude that the product isn't very good for the symptom of flatulence. Trials like this, whether looking at food supplements or drugs, are judged on how much better the active product performed compared to placebo. So the placebo *is* an annoyance for people trying to show that their product is effective. But on the other hand, the placebo effect is amazing – people can improve their symptoms by simply taking an inert pill!

For drug companies, the placebo effect might well be a nuisance, but for medical practice, it might be useful: it could help people get better.

Why do placebos work?

Placebo effects have been explained by several mechanisms.

- When people are given a treatment, they expect there to be some clinical improvement. The fact that they generally *do* improve shows the power of mind over matter.
- Placebo effects work better when the treatment is endorsed by an expert (such as a GP) – so again, a belief that the treatment will work is important.
- It may also be due to simple Pavlovian conditioning (also called classical conditioning). The Russian physiologist Ivan Pavlov experimented by feeding dogs and ringing a bell at the same time. After a number of trials, the dogs associated the ringing bell with food and, at the sound of the bell, they salivated even without food. So the sound of the bell elicited a physiological response.

Here is another example of conditioning, relevant to people with disease. Ciclosprin (also known as cyclosporine) is an immunosuppressant drug that is given to people who have had an organ transplant so that the body doesn't reject the organ. If people are given ciclosporin and a flavoured drink on several occasions, then later, when given the flavoured drink alone, their immune functions are suppressed – the body reacts as if they had taken the ciclosporin (biological measurements were taken to determine this). So the immune system can be conditioned to respond to tastes – and smells.

Say that you take a drug that affects the immune system – there is an immune response caused by ingesting the drug. Imagine that every time you are given the drug, you are given a particular fragrance to smell. Once this has happened a few times, when you smell the fragrance, your body will react by giving the same immune response, without you having to ingest the drug. Isn't that amazing?

Neuroimaging studies in placebo trials

Brain imaging has also shown neurobiological responses to treatment with a placebo that are similar to those seen in patients treated with an active agent. Studies have shown that if you expect the treatment to work, the placebo effects will be increased, but even with no expectations of benefit, the placebo still works.

Positron emission tomography (PET) scans are used to produce three-dimensional images of the brain and inside of the body. These images can help diagnose diseases such as cancer. In a study in 2004, patients with IBS had PET scans before and after receiving a placebo for three weeks. They were told that the pills, which were inactive substances, might reduce their symptoms. PET scans showed activity in a particular part of the brain that was related to positive expectations about the placebo treatment, thus showing that positive expectations are important.

A study in 2008 investigated the PET scans of people with Parkinson's disease. Parkinson's disease is characterized by a progressive loss of dopamine, which causes problems with movement. When the patients were given a placebo pill to improve their symptoms, the PET scans showed a release of the dopamine in the brain. The amount of dopamine produced was greater in those patients who believed the placebo was working than in those who didn't. These effects are neuropsychobiological phenomena – the effects are not only psychological, they are due to an interaction between neurological, psychological and biological processes.

Nocebo effects

The opposite of the placebo effect (the nocebo effect) traditionally refers to any treatment that has adverse effects, and 'nocebo' means 'I shall harm'. The way we think about nocebos has expanded, so that now the effect relates not just to a pill that is expected to have an adverse effect, but to the psychosocial context around the patient and the treatment, such as the words spoken to the patient by the therapist or doctor, which will affect the therapeutic outcome.

Suggestions of no effect or a negative effect in medicine lead to a worse outcome. Even a GP saying, 'This will work' has a different effect from, 'This might work.' Negative diagnosis (for example, if you have cancer and in a person your age the prognosis is poor) can lead to symptom worsening. Negative expectations can lead to the nocebo effect with consequent adverse neuropsychological effects. Health warnings and those long lists of side effects given in patient leaflets may adversely affect some people.

In some nocebo experiments, no pills or treatment have been given, but instead the participants are given negative verbal suggestions only. Negative expectations can result in more pain, and several brain regions have been found to be activated during the anticipation of pain. These are called nocebo-related effects, because no inert substance has been given. In one study, post-operative patients received morphine for 48 hours, then their morphine was interrupted (switched off for a while). Some patients were told that the morphine was stopped and some were not told. The pain increase was larger when they were told about the interruption than when they were not told. This has clinical implications. If therapy has to be interrupted, then telling the patient might induce a nocebo response. Other studies have confirmed these effects.

This is concrete evidence that the mind can affect the brain and body. These mind processes are called mentalistic variables. They consist of thoughts, feelings, beliefs and intentions. These mentalistic variables (the mind) influence the function of the brain. As we said in Chapter 1, some people believe these mentalistic processes are just by-products of brain activity. However, placebo and nocebo effects seem to contradict this view of the mind–brain–body.

You have seen from just a few studies discussed above (and there are many more) that mentalistic processes can influence your brain and your body. Many studies show that negative mentalistic processes affect health. For instance, depression, anxiety, pessimism and other such states increase inflammation and give you a greater likelihood of illness. We have already seen in Chapter 4 that stress and depression do this. Anger, hostility and pessimism work in similar ways. If you are cynical and suspicious, and tend to see the world in a pessimistic way, this increases the likelihood of heart disease. Distrust and hostility also is associated with more inflammation and a greater risk of chronic illnesses, such as diabetes.

Of course, we know that such mentalistic variables affect other aspects of life as well. So people who are angry and hostile are more likely to have fewer friends and therefore fewer sources of social support. You have probably heard of the benefits of marriage for couples. It has been found that for men, marriage reduces the risk of early death by 500 per cent, but for women it is 50 per cent. Of course it is not as simple as this. Just being married is not enough to ensure a long and happy life. Women who remained silent in marital conflicts were four times more likely to die than those who didn't. And marital conflict unsurprisingly has a negative impact on health – it increases the risk of heart disease, especially for women. Trauma – whether early violent or sexual abuse, maltreatment, or wars or other disasters – also has long-lasting adverse effects on people, not just psychological effects but also physiological ones, such as higher levels of proinflammatory cytokines and other measures of inflammation. However, people differ in the ways they think about such events and make sense of them. The way we think about awful things that have happened to us – whether we dwell on them and keep going over them (rumination) or whether we try to cope with such feelings by talking about them, joining self-help groups or going to counselling – can make a big difference to the mind and the body. Psychologists have found that the way we perceive or appraise awful events matters in long-term coping.

Optimism and positive thinking

How would you describe yourself? Psychologists think of optimism and pessimism as dispositional traits – that is, people tend towards either one or the other. Studies show that being an optimist helps you to cope with your illness much better than if you are a pessimist. In part, this is due to the fact that optimists tend to try to find ways of coping with their symptoms, and in so doing, find more effective coping strategies. They also try to improve their health by following good practices, such as diet and exercise. This doesn't mean that positive thinking will cure your illness – if only it were that easy! But psychologists have found that people who persevere in being optimistic despite their illness adapt more effectively to their illness and have better physical and psychological health.

Swedish researchers studied the strategies that women with FMS (all of whom were still in work) used to help themselves. Their strategies were to try to enjoy life (despite their illness), to ensure they took care of themselves, to think positively, to use their pain as a guide in what to do and what not to do, and to learn and be knowledgeable about FMS. These were *conscious* strategies – that is, the subjects made a conscious effort to remain positive. So these women with FMS tried to focus on the aspects of their lives that were good, and they recast their thoughts. For example, when they had to take sick leave, instead of thinking of this as a negative, they focused on the positive aspects (more time to read or to take walks). They thought about eating well, avoiding unnecessary stress and doing everything to ensure that their bodies functioned as well as possible. They chose which activities to focus on, bearing in mind how their energy levels were that day. In other words, they prioritized what they could do.

Choosing techniques to help yourself when you are ill is sometimes very difficult indeed, but studies show that doing something ('doing' can simply be sitting down and meditating or similar) is important. Making a conscious effort to do something like this (even if you are sceptical that such techniques will work) is better than doing nothing. Psychologists have found that negative emotions stimulate overproduction of proinflammatory cytokines and that even people with no illness who perceived minor life events in a negative way had more physical health problems.

This doesn't mean that you must suppress negative emotions, because suppressing feelings is bad for you too. Negative emotions are part of life, but the way forward is not to focus on them and not to ruminate about them. Your life is changed when you have a chronic or long-term illness, the illness changes you, and when you first have the illness, naturally you want to fight against it. You want your old life back. But accepting that you now have such an illness doesn't mean you have to be passive and give up. You can accept you have this illness *now* (and maybe it will last for months, or even years) but people with the illnesses such as the ones we talk about in this book get better, and cope better over time. In other words, you recover – it's just that recovery isn't going back to where you were before you had the chronic illness. Maybe you can no longer go for long bike rides, or run a marathon, or go on a cruise or even on a long walk. But there are other things in life that you can do and that will give you pleasure – you just have to find out what these are. One study found that women with FMS grieved for their lost health, but that accepting their situation helped them to cope, and that social support from their families helped them too.

Can you influence the course of your illness by changing the way you think about your illness? And does it depend on the type of illness you have? The answers are yes. Some illnesses are controllable by self-care, at least to some extent. Although you might have CFS/ME or IBS, for instance, certain lifestyle choices might affect your symptoms, negatively or positively. Pacing is important in CFS/ME, and this will help you control your symptoms, although people vary in the extent to which this will help, depending on their stage of illness, the social support they have, whether they go to work, and so on. Making a decision to go jogging because you feel you are better (even though you are not) could lead to a relapse. For CFS/ME and the other illnesses that we discuss, taking time out to relax and meditate and visualizing yourself being healthy should help – as we know, these relaxation responses (regulated by the parasympathetic nervous system) are the opposite of those of the sympathetic nervous system (which prepares the body for fight and flight). When you are practising relaxation techniques, the sympathetic nervous system is unable to stimulate the release of stress hormones and increase the heart rate, because the two systems are antagonistic to each other.

> I was having migraines every week. I know that migraine is a physical illness, and so when I was advised to do relaxation techniques and meditation, I didn't think they would work. My doctor said that meditation could reduce my heart rate, so I bought some meditation CDs, and decided to see whether they helped. I didn't like the CDs, but once I understood what to do I meditated on my own. I took my pulse rate before the meditation, and again after the meditation. I didn't really think it would work. But after a few weeks of meditation, my pulse rate was lower, and I think the migraines were not as bad, or maybe I just coped better with them. Anyway, I decided it didn't matter why it worked, as long as it helped. I try to meditate a few times each week during my lunch break, just to calm myself down. (NW, with migraine)

When illnesses are, at least in part, controllable, then positive beliefs and optimism can improve your health. These are the illnesses we discuss in this book, and research shows that the way you think about your illness can affect its progression.

Remember the quotation from Professor Beauregard at the start of Chapter 1? Professor Beauregard is a world-leading neuroscientist from the University of Montreal. He has more than 100 publications (including work on the placebo and nocebo effects) in the fields of neuroscience, psychology and psychiatry. His work has led him to believe that the mind is not identical to the brain. Indeed, he believes that the mind (consisting of mentalistic variables) is real and can influence, and even change, the brain.

In this chapter we have discussed just some of the amazing findings in relation to these effects. We know from the discussions in previous chapters in relation to psychoneuroimmunology that the brain and the immune system communicate with each other, just as the brain communicates with the digestive system. In fact, really all these systems are like pieces of one amazing communicative jigsaw; they are all linked together and all communicate with one another.

If the mind can affect the workings of, or even change, the brain, is it possible for you to use your mind to affect your immune system? We already know that stress, depression and anxiety can affect your immune system (see Chapter 4). If you have any of the illnesses that we focus on in this book, or similar illnesses, your immune system is likely to be affected. Can you affect your immune system, say, by guided imagery or visualization? For instance, would imagining your natural killer cells arising from their slumber and helping to fight viruses actually affect the natural killer cells? And if natural killer cells are affected, is it simply a result of relaxation as you carry out your imagining, or is it something more fundamental – that is, is your mind really communicating with the natural killer cells?

One study looked at groups of students taking examinations, which can be very stressful. There were three groups: a control group (who took the examinations but didn't receive any intervention in the form of imagery or relaxation), an immune imagery group and a relaxation group. In the immune imagery group, participants were taught to use imagery to improve the immune system, by envisaging increases in natural killer cells and lymphocytes, as well as thinking about white blood cells in the form of sharks, devouring viruses or bacteria. In the relaxation group participants were taught to relax and think of peace, happiness and tranquillity. The researchers looked at how many students from each group fell ill during the examination period. The numbers of the students who fell ill were highest in the control group, and lowest in the immune imagery group, the relaxation group being midway. These were important differences.

Another study looked at patients with breast cancer, who either had autogenic training, which is a relaxation technique, or guided-imagery only. Both investigations increased natural killer cells counts after two months.

> If the state of physical distress can depress the immune system and decrease the level of personal health, then interventions designed to reduce distress should relieve pressure on the immune system and allow it to function more effectively, thereby leading to better personal health.   (Donaldson, 2000, p. 118)

There are many scientific studies carried out to determine whether immunity improves as a result of guided imagery. The studies show that using guided imagery to think about specific types of cells (such as white cells or natural killer cells) can change the activity of those cells. Donaldson believes that this is because every thought has a physiological response, so that thoughts about specific body activities activate the neurones related to that activity. So imagining that the natural killer cells are awakening and fighting a virus, or imagining that the cells are simply moving around in a surveillance mode, *will* have an effect on the immune system.

Other studies have found that hypnosis, guided imagery and relaxation improve depression and stress and reduce blood pressure. These techniques can reduce cortisol levels and help immune-related disorders.

As with the placebo effect, we don't really understand the complex ways in which mentalistic techniques (such as positive affirmations and mental imagery) affect us. However, we do know now that the brain is not static – it changes over time and throughout life. It changes as a result of life experiences and the way in which we make sense of those experiences. It changes as a result of the thoughts we have.

Are you sceptical about this? Can the mind give rise to a physiological response? Imagine cutting a lemon in half and then squeezing the juice into your mouth. What happens? You are probably aware of salivating. Since you are only imagining drinking the juice of a lemon, it is obvious that it is your mind that has affected the physiological process of salivating. Remember that the immune system can be conditioned in a similar way.

Summary and conclusion

By describing some of the scientific studies on placebos, nocebos and mentalistic techniques such as guided imagery, we have shown you the ways in which our minds and brains can affect biological processes. Remember, you have nothing to lose by trying these techniques – many lead to the relaxation response, lowering your blood pressure and reducing anxiety. They certainly won't have harmful side effects! There is evidence that, although your illness may be physical, you can improve your life. These improvements may be small, it's true, but even small improvements help. We give you information about treatments and techniques in Chapters 6 and 7.

6

Treatments

Manage the whole disorder, be realistic.
(Dr Anish Bahra, neurologist, speaking at the 'Migraine and Me'
conference, Royal Society of Medicine, London, April 2013)

This chapter outlines a number of suggested treatments and management strategies that have been used in the long-term conditions covered in this book. This is simply a review of available information and should not be a replacement for medical advice. However, the suggestions we give may help you to be aware of the various options and also to gain appropriate treatment.

Medications

As different drugs can be beneficial to different conditions, we take each invisible illness in turn for this sub-section.

IBS

A number of medications can be used to manage the symptoms of IBS. These will not resolve the underlying problem but can help with constipation, diarrhoea, pain, and so on. Anti-spasmodic medicines such as mebeverine and therapeutic peppermint oil can diminish pain and cramping by relaxing the muscles in the digestive system. Like all drugs, there can be side effects (although these are rare). For example, peppermint oil can cause heartburn.

Perhaps surprisingly, anti-depressants can also be used if anti-spasmodic medications have not been successful at reducing pain and cramping. Two types of anti-depressants can be used to treat IBS – tricyclic anti-depressants (most commonly amitriptyline) and selective serotonin reuptake inhibitors (SSRIs) such as citalopram, fluoxetine and paroxetine. Anti-depressants work by altering some of the chemicals in the brain known as neurotransmitters, which are released by nerve cells to send signals to other nerve cells. Tricyclic anti-depressants raise the levels of the serotonin and noradrenaline, and SSRIs increase serotonin, known as the 'happiness hormone' because it plays an important part in mood regulation. People with depression have been shown to have fewer serotonin receptors, which is why SSRIs can help with depression in some people. Tricyclic anti-depressants can have side effects (dry mouth, constipation, blurred vision and drowsiness), although these usually lessen after a few days of taking the medicine. They are not suitable if you have some cardiac problems. The side effects of SSRIs include blurred vision, diarrhoea or constipation, and dizziness. If the side effects do not go away, your doctor may suggest a different anti-depressant to see if that works better for you. For tricyclic anti-depressants to work, they must be taken consistently as they will only provide symptom relief as the body starts to get used to them, usually three to four weeks after starting the course. They are not a 'quick fix' and should be supervised by your doctor.

For diarrhoea, anti-motility medicines such as loperamide may help. These work by reducing the rate at which food progresses through the digestive system by slowing down the muscle contractions in the bowel. However, loperamide can cause abdominal cramps and bloating, dizziness, drowsiness and skin rashes, and it should not be taken by pregnant women.

For constipation, bulk-forming laxatives can be used. These are fibre supplements and work in the same manner as fibre that you eat by enabling the retention of fluid in the stool, which makes them easier to pass. However, it is vital that sufficient water is consumed when taking this type of laxative, otherwise the bowels can become blocked. Also, bloating and wind can be side effects of laxatives so it is important to start on a low dose and increase gradually until one or two soft stools are passed every one or two days. Bulk-forming laxatives should not be taken at bedtime as you need to drink a fair amount of water when taking them to avoid a blockage. If you take them at night, you will not be drinking enough water over the next eight hours, and therefore you might actually find it very difficult to have a bowel movement. When bowel movements are so hard that you cannot expel your stool, then you may have faecal impaction, in which case, you should seek advice from your doctor.

Migraine

Over-the-counter painkillers such as paracetamol and aspirin can be used to manage the pain associated with a migraine (instructions on the packets should be followed and people with stomach problems, such as a peptic ulcer, liver problems or kidney problems should not take aspirin). Painkillers are usually most effective when taken at the first signs of a migraine attack, even if pain is not the first symptom, as this will give the medicine more time to be absorbed into the bloodstream. It is not recommended to wait until the migraine becomes worse before you take painkillers because, by this point, it is often too late for the medicine to have a beneficial effect. Soluble tablets (dissolved in water) are absorbed into the bloodstream more quickly than normal pills and can be used if you find tablets hard to swallow. Suppositories (tablets or capsules inserted into the rectum (the back passage)) can also be used if other types of painkillers cause nausea or vomiting. Anti-inflammatory medications, such as ibuprofen (available over the counter) or diclofenac, naproxen and tolfenamic acid (prescription only) can also help some people with migraines. However, there is a very important point – painkillers can actually cause migraines and headaches themselves. Such headaches are known as medication-overuse headaches and are commonly associated with the painkillers codeine and ibuprofen. Therefore, it is important to get the balance right in medication use, and you may need the support of a GP (possibly one with a special interest in headache and migraine) or a specialist clinic. Do ask your GP about this if you are finding it hard to know when to take pain relief.

Triptans can also help to relieve the symptoms of migraine. They do not work in the same way as painkillers. They do not stop pain signals going to the brain but rather they narrow the blood vessels around the brain by making them contract. It is believed this process helps to decrease symptoms by reversing the dilation or widening of the blood vessels that is associated with migraine. Some types of triptans can be bought over the counter, such as sumatriptan, although others need a prescription from the doctor. Triptans come in tablet and nasal forms and also as injections. They do not work for everyone, and some types work better for some people than others, so it is good to discuss this with your GP to find the right medicine for your migraines.

Anti-sickness medicines can be used to treat migraine, even if nausea is not a symptom. These should be taken at the first sign of the migraine and can be taken alongside painkillers. In fact, some tablets that can be purchased at the pharmacy are combination medicines, containing both pain relief and anti-sickness components. Pharmacists are often very knowledgeable about these medicines so it can be worth discussing your symptoms to see which type may be best for you. However, the dosage in these over-the-counter drugs may not be sufficient to prevent a migraine attack in some people, so it may be better to take the painkillers and anti-sickness medicines separately, which allows for more control over dosage.

For menstrual migraine, a specific type of migraine, as previously discussed, hormonal treatment can be helpful. The combined oral contraceptive pill and some types of contraceptive implants and devices can help to prevent attacks. Oestrogen patches that are placed on the skin three days before the start of your period and are kept on for seven days can also be used to treat this type of migraine. These patches are similar in size and appearance to nicotine patches. These treatments may help with migraine attacks by stabilizing the drop in oestrogen, which can be associated with peak migraine episodes.

FMS

As in migraine, pain is a core symptom in FMS and hence painkillers are often prescribed and recommended by your doctor or pharmacist. Paracetamol is the most common over-the-counter pain relief used in FMS but if this is not strong enough, a doctor may prescribe codeine or tramadol. Tramadol appears to be effective for some people with FMS, who report an increase in their daily activities after taking it. However, the side effects of tramadol can include diarrhoea and severe fatigue, and withdrawal symptoms if it is stopped.

If sleep disturbance is an issue for you, over-the-counter remedies based on natural products such as valerian may be recommended, or your doctor may prescribe sleeping tablets, in addition to sleep hygiene advice (see Chapter 7).

Muscle stiffness and spasms may be helped by muscle relaxant drugs, which can also aid sleep because they have sleep-inducing, sedative effects. (Care should be taken when driving if using these medicines.)

Anti-convulsant (anti-seizure) medications, which are used in epilepsy, may also help with the symptoms of FMS. Pregabalin (often the brand called Lyrica) is the most frequently prescribed type of anti-convulsant in FMS. This does not mean that you might have epilepsy, but simply that this particular drug has been shown through research studies to improve the symptoms of FMS in up to 40 per cent of people. However, like all medications, pregabalin can cause side effects, the most common being dry mouth, dizziness, blurred vision, weight gain and gastrointestinal complaints such as constipation, nausea and vomiting. Side effects should be discussed with your doctor.

Anti-depressants are often recommended for people with FMS, but not as a treatment for depression (although you may have symptoms of depression, and this is completely understandable) but to boost the amount of neurotransmitters in the brain. Neurotransmitters, including serotonin, noradrenaline and dopamine, are chemicals that carry signals or messages to and from the brain. Some scientists believe that low levels of neurotransmitters may be partly responsible for the symptoms of FMS and therefore, if the levels are increased, symptoms may diminish. There are various types of anti-depressants and the type you are prescribed will depend on your individual symptoms and their severity. In addition to tricyclic anti-depressants and SSRIs, serotonin–noradrenaline reuptake inhibitors, such as duloxetine, may be recommended to raise levels of serotonin and noradrenaline.

Finally, the medicines pramipexole and tropisetron also act on brain neurotransmitters and may be used in FMS. (Interestingly, pramipexole is also used to relieve restless leg syndrome, a condition that is sometimes reported in those with FMS.)

CFS/ME

If pain is a symptom of your CFS/ME, the over-the-counter medicines discussed above may offer some relief, and your doctor can prescribe stronger medications if the pain is severe.

Anti-depressants may also help to relieve pain and sleep problems. The most common anti-depressant prescribed for those with CFS/ME is amitriptyline.

Nausea in CFS/ME may be helped with an anti-emetic, which is a type of drug often used for motion sickness and morning sickness.

Anti-viral medications are not commonly prescribed for CFS/ME, nor are medicines for thyroid dysfunction, (e.g. thyroxin), although there is still a debate about whether these would be appropriate for some people with CFS/ME. Currently, there is research being conducted into the drug rituximab, and a group of Norwegian oncologists have found that it reduced symptoms in some people with CFS/ME. (This was a surprising finding because it was not a part of the original study, which was about the cancer Hodgkin's lymphoma, but some of the patients had CFS/ME prior to developing cancer.) Rituximab strips away a type of cell called the B cell, which makes antibodies that fight off viruses and other foreign invaders. B cells also produce autoantibodies, which attack the body's own tissues in autoimmune conditions such as rheumatoid arthritis. This has led some commentators to question whether CFS/ME is an autoimmune disease. More research needs to be carried out in this area but it is an interesting direction for research studies and may offer more comprehensive treatments for this debilitating condition.

Ménière's disease

Prochlorperazine or anti-histamines (such as cinnarizine, cyclizine or promethazine teoclate) can be prescribed for 7 to 14 days to treat vertigo, nausea and vomiting. It is useful to have a supply of these handy to tackle the symptoms as soon as they start.

Prochlorperazine acts by blocking dopamine receptors in the brain. Side effects can include drowsiness, tremors or shaking and involuntary body and facial movements. If vomiting is a symptom of your Ménière's disease, a type of prochlorperazine known as Buccastem can be used. This is placed in the mouth, between the gums and the cheek, where it dissolves and is then absorbed into the body. In a very severe attack, your doctor may wish to inject the prochlorperazine directly into your bloodstream to counteract the vertigo, dizziness, nausea and vomiting that you may experience. Side effects of anti-histamines include sleepiness, headaches and stomach upset.

In very extreme attacks in Ménière's disease, it may be necessary to go into hospital for hydration via an intravenous drip, but this is rare.

To prevent attacks, the medication betahistine may be advised. Betahistine works by reducing the pressure in the inner eye, which is thought to cause some of the symptoms in Ménière's disease, specifically vertigo, tinnitus and hearing loss, although the jury is still out regarding whether betahistine is definitely effective. Your doctor can prescribe this medication and will need to decide how long you should take it for. This can be anywhere from a few weeks up to a year. Side effects include skin rashes, headaches and stomach upset.

In addition to general dietary advice (see Chapter 7), a specialist diet that excludes salt can be beneficial in Ménière's disease. The theory behind this diet is that salts alter the fluid in the inner ear, and therefore maintaining a low-salt diet may help to manage symptoms. People have also reported that some foods, including chocolate, nuts and red wine, are triggers for symptoms, so it could be worth keeping a food diary to try to pinpoint any food triggers you may have. Caffeinated drinks like coffee, tea and cola may also be triggers, so keep an eye out for these if you are having symptoms.

Because tinnitus can be such an intrusive symptom, there are particular treatments for this symptom alone, such as sound therapy. Tinnitus can seem much worse in quiet environments, and sound therapy lessens the difference between tinnitus sounds and background sounds so that the tinnitus becomes less intrusive. Some people find cognitive behavioural therapy (CBT; see below) and relaxation techniques (see Chapter 7) helpful.

If hearing loss is a problem, hearing aids can be used to reduce the sensitivity to loud sounds and increase your ability to pick up low-pitched sounds. (See Useful addresses for details of how to find a local audiologist.)

MdDS

Because MdDS is such a rare condition and so few research studies have been carried out on people with MdDS, it is unclear which treatments are best for the condition. We do know, however, that the drugs used to treat Ménière's disease do not seem to help in MdDS.

Benzodiazepines (such as clonazepam) appear to provide the best symptomatic relief. A low dose is usually prescribed because higher doses are not normally effective. Benzodiazepines do not help everyone with MdDS, but when they do work, sleep is improved and daytime balance is better. The main drawback is sedation (sleepiness) and the possibility of addiction.

The anti-depressant SSRIs can also help with the symptoms of MdDS, and some doctors suggest taking these regularly, with benzodiazepines when needed for symptom flare-ups.

Other treatments

Cognitive behavioural therapy (CBT)

Like the strategies above, CBT is not a 'cure' for invisible illnesses but may help in coping with these conditions. CBT is used in a wide range of illnesses, including those with an underlying disease process such as cancer, multiple sclerosis and rheumatoid arthritis, and also in disorders without a known cause, such as the ones in this book. Some people may feel that they do not want to try CBT because it is a psychological technique, but CBT is usually offered to reduce some of the anxiety and low mood that can be experienced when faced with the severe restrictions on life as mentioned in Chapter 3. CBT works by breaking thought patterns that can make us feel anxious and depressed. CBT cannot, in and of itself, eradicate the physical symptoms of long-term illness, but it may reduce stress and the impact on the HPA axis (see Chapters 2 and 4).

> I was a bit reluctant to try CBT, if I'm honest. I thought my doctor thought I was just some mad old bat and wanted me out of his office! But my daughter said I should give it a go, which I did, with reservations, mind you. I went for six weeks and did all the homework that the psychologist lady said and in the end, I found I could stop being so angry about being ill. I wouldn't say it's cured me, no, but it's certainly helped me get more out of life and I am thankful to them, and my daughter, for that.
> (JK, with IBS)

Graded exercise therapy (GET)

GET uses some of the techniques of CBT but, in addition, gradual increases in activities are built into treatment. GET is most often used for disorders like FMS and CFS/ME where the amount of activity has been significantly reduced due to ill health.

GET should be supervised by a trained professional such as an occupational therapist to ensure that a 'boom and bust' pattern does not develop. Boom and bust means trying to do too much when feeling a bit better, which often leads to a relapse (the bust). This can be incredibly distressing and can lead to worsening symptoms. By first getting to grips with a person's baseline level of activity (what can be done comfortably without causing additional symptoms), the therapist can develop a structured programme. Within this programme there will be set goals that can be related to the length of a particular activity or the intensity of a task. For example, an end-goal may be to be able to walk to the shops, but this will be broken down into steps that may start initially by walking across the front room. The speed at which these goals are obtained is completely to do with the person's unique situation and it might take weeks, months or even years to accomplish the end-goals, which is why it is important to do GET with a professional who can help identify manageable interim steps and maintain motivation.

However, it should be noted that not everyone thinks GET is a good treatment for disorders such as CFS/ME. Recently, researchers have been looking at some possible physiological problems in people with CFS/ME that could explain their symptoms, rather than it being down to deconditioning or fear of activity. If these theories are supported, it may in fact provide the reason why some people feel that GET makes their condition worse. Two of the largest UK-based CFS/ME charities, the ME Association and Action for ME, carried out surveys that asked respondents about treatments they had tried. The first survey found that 33 per cent of people said that GET made them much worse (23 per cent said they felt slightly worse, 21 per cent reported no change in symptoms, 19 per cent improved and 3 per cent had improved greatly). The second survey had even higher negative responses, with 60 per cent of people stating that their condition had worsened following a course of GET (22 per cent of respondents reported improvements after GET). These surveys were not carried out in a 'scientific' fashion so should perhaps be viewed with caution (for example, it may be that people who had bad experiences with GET were more likely to engage in such a survey), but it is useful to know others' experiences when thinking about which treatments you may want to embark upon.

Physiotherapy

Balance problems are a common complaint in both Ménière's disease and MdDS, and physiotherapy can help by teaching you vestibular rehabilitation techniques. Giddiness and vertigo can also be symptoms for those with CFS/ME and FMS, although they are less commonly mentioned by patients (perhaps because people are not explicitly asked about balance problems in these disorders). Hence physiotherapy may be appropriate for many long-term conditions, not just the ones with obvious balance issues, so if you have such symptoms please do ask your doctor for advice.

As the signals from the inner ear can cause disorientation, the physiotherapist will show you how to rely on signals from other parts of the body such as the eyes, ankles, legs and neck to maintain balance. However, physiotherapy is usually offered only in the mid-to-late stages of Ménière's disease, when the severe vertigo attacks have stopped but when there are still difficulties in balance. Vestibular rehabilitation (sometimes known as Cawthorne–Cooksey exercises) has also been said to help with some of the symptoms of MdDS, so a referral from your GP to a physiotherapist may help with the balance issues associated with MdDS.

Surgery

In very severe cases of Ménière's disease (about 10 per cent of the total) surgery may be required. However, surgery is only an option if all other treatments have failed. Three types of surgery can be used for Ménière's disease:

- non-destructive surgery
- selectively destructive surgery
- destructive surgery.

There is very little evidence from research about the benefits of surgery in Ménière's disease, so this is something that would have to be thought about very carefully with your ENT specialist.

Surgery is not recommended for any of the other disorders in this book.

Complementary and alternative medicine

There are countless approaches in complementary and alternative medicine (CAM) and many do not have enough evidence to be recommended for the long-term conditions in this book. If you are tempted to try CAM, find out if there is some persuasive scientific evidence for its effectiveness – this is more than testimonials and success stories on websites; rather there should be published studies in respectable scientific journals that have used research tools to evaluate the technique properly. Seeking out this information yourself when feeling dreadful can be overwhelming, so you can simply ask the practitioner what evidence there is for the approach. Anyone who is confident that the techniques are evidence-based (all this means is that the research studies have been conducted and shown good results) will be happy to share with you the published papers and explain the result to you. This can save you a great deal of time, money and energy when you may be severely lacking the latter two! At present, the Advertising Standards Agency has been clamping down on health-care providers to ensure that they do not over-state their claims. This is a positive move that should help people to be aware of which therapies work and which therapies have yet to be shown to help.

However, there are some types of CAM that have been tested rigorously and can be recommended for our invisible illnesses.

Acupuncture

Acupuncture is a type of traditional Chinese medicine in which the practitioner inserts fine needles into various points on the body (called acupuncture points) in order to stimulate certain areas. We now believe that acupuncture works by reducing inflammation, encouraging the release of endorphins (yet another type of neurotransmitter that can block the release of pain signals) and calming the mind. It is a safe treatment. The only side effects that have been reported are mild pain at the place where the needles are inserted and lethargy (tiredness), both of which are short-lasting.

When there are many research studies published on a topic and we want to know what the overall picture is for whether a treatment works or not, a type of analysis called meta-analysis may be carried out. The statistics for this analytic technique are quite complex but the end-result is an estimate of the treatment's effectiveness across all the studies. These studies, when taken together, can contain hundreds of research participants. This is important because very large studies are often too expensive and arduous to carry out. A group of researchers recently used this method to look at whether acupuncture is a beneficial therapy for FMS.

The researchers found nine studies that looked at acupuncture as a treatment for FMS, which had a total of 395 participants, and collated the information from these studies. They found that in comparison to no treatment or standard treatment, acupuncture was better at reducing pain and stiffness in people with FMS. When looking at different types of acupuncture, electro-acupuncture (which involves a small electric current being passed between pairs of acupuncture needles) was better than manual acupuncture (without electrical stimulation) for the relief of pain and stiffness and also for improving general well-being, sleep and fatigue. Therefore, from looking at the information across a number of studies, it can be concluded that acupuncture is beneficial for some people with FMS. (Of course not everyone will have good results, as with any other treatment, but it may be worth a try based on the evidence.)

Perhaps a lot of people are put off by the needles but they're not like the needles when the nurse takes blood – they're tiny and you hardly feel a thing. I would say it's more like having some nice facial or massage, as I left my appointments feeling floaty and relaxed. I had eight sessions at first and now I go back for top-ups and also I just like it, and I like Clare who does it and I think it has helped me with my pain. (EG, with FMS)

Hypnotherapy

During a session of hypnotherapy, the practitioner will help you to reach a hypnotic state by using techniques such as guided imagery or progressive muscle relaxation. This process is known as hypnotic induction. A hypnotic state is like being in deep relaxation in which you are in control and quite aware of what's going on around you but new ideas and information can be processed at the subconscious level. It is at this level of consciousness that the fight or flight response resides – that is, it happens automatically and is apparently beyond our control. Therefore, hypnotherapy may help to control the stress response but also other habituated or learned responses such as phobias, as described below.

I happened to meet a practitioner at my daughter's playgroup and we got talking about my phobia of spiders. He said he could cure that in half an hour. I had been raised in a Baptist church environment and was always warned off anything to do with hypnosis, and when I told him about this caution, he said he'd been raised in the same way but the reason he trained in hypnosis was to help people. So I bit the bullet and went for it. After one short session, my spider phobia was gone, ending years of trouble! I saw him a few more times for other reasons, and then one day after having another panic attack I wondered if he might be able to help with anxiety. Of course, he said he could. I explained the severity of the problem – how I couldn't bear to get on a motorway or drive over 50 m.p.h., how I would wake in the night shaking, how I would find myself caught in an anxiety loop every time I experienced a strange twitch or other symptom. Two sessions later, I was a changed man. Back in the car, making long motorway journeys without the tight chest and pounding head. Brushing aside those twitches and, essentially, just not having that anxiety to bring me further down and accentuate the negatives of CFS/ME. I've held this belief for some time – that anxiety is one of the crucial factors in worsening CFS/ME. The anxiety loop seems to amplify everything, like a sound that just gets louder and louder, pushing you lower and lower. Breaking that loop has made such a difference – a life-changing difference indeed. Although I am by no means recovered from CFS/ME, it has become much easier to live with, and I find I take a much more rational approach to it now. It has empowered me to remain positive – a major factor in dealing with any illness, I say. The techniques my practitioner used were barely noticeable. At no point was I 'under', or feeling like I had lost any control. As he explained, we spend much of our lives in a trance – driving a familiar journey, brushing our teeth even, and we are open to suggestion during these times. It's how billboard advertising works. Being in a passive state is natural, really. So although he was working a certain 'magic' with me at the time, there was no odd sensation or discomfort. It was pleasant, enjoyable even and, most importantly, effective!   (CR, with CFS/ME)

Hypnotherapy has been studied a great deal in people with IBS. In 2006, a group of researchers carried out a systematic review of 15 studies of hypnotherapy in IBS. They found that, overall, people who had hypnotherapy saw improvements in IBS symptoms, compared to those having other treatments such as psychotherapy, those having non-treatment such as symptom-monitoring and those on a waiting list. In addition, people who had undergone hypnotherapy also had better ratings of quality of life after treatment, and their levels of anxiety and depression decreased. These findings appear long-lasting, up to two to five years. Interestingly, many of the studies reviewed used slightly different forms of hypnotherapy. Some used techniques to increase progressive muscle relaxation, some simply used hypnotic induction, while others used 'gut-directed' hypnotherapy. Gut-directed hypnotherapy involves first explaining to the patient the way in which the gut works and what may be triggering the symptoms of IBS. While under hypnosis, the patient learns how to control gut activity by using techniques such as imagery and hand warmth on the abdomen. It can be used at home.

Also in 2006, a group of researchers and doctors in the north of England used gut-directed hypnotherapy for people who did not find relief with any of the more conventional treatments. Three months after the treatment, people who had the hypnotherapy reported less pain, diarrhoea and overall symptoms than people who were using conventional treatment alone. Notably, people who used the hypnotic skills were less likely to need medication to control their symptoms, which is an important finding when thinking about mind over matter (see Chapter 5).

Summary and conclusion

This chapter has outlined some of the treatment alternatives for the long-term conditions we are interested in. Although the conventional options like pharmacology may differ between the illnesses, all the CAM techniques aim to work at the mind–body interface and so could be beneficial for the entire range of conditions, although we won't know this for sure until more research is carried out. The next chapter looks at some more things you can do to help control your illness and take back your life.

7

Self-help:
other ways to improve your life

One person said to me to try this and that and then another said, 'You've got to do this, it totally cured me!' There are so many things out there and it is hard to know which ones to try but, in my view, the basics things, things that I hadn't even realized were messed up, have been the ones that have helped me the most. (DD, with migraine)

Following on from the previous chapter that looked at treatments for which you need to see a doctor, nurse, physiotherapist, psychologist or other type of health-care professional, this chapter aims to give you some techniques that you can use yourself. Most of the ideas here are about creating and maintaining an even keel in life, which can help to reduce stress and improve sleep and result in a better quality of daily living.

Diary-keeping

First, it is vital that you get the right diagnosis from your doctor. To do this, it is important to help your GP or specialist to disentangle the myriad of symptoms that can be experienced with invisible illness. Keeping a detailed symptom diary can help enormously. There are some symptom-specific diaries – for example, headache diaries – and these can be daily, weekly or monthly. Headache diaries generally ask when the pain started and about its severity and any other associated symptoms, such as nausea, aura and sensitivity to light, sound or smell. There are also fatigue diaries and diaries for the symptoms of CFS/ME, IBS and FMS, and your consultant may even have a version that he or she would like you to use (Figure 6).

In this age of technology, many smartphones have applications that act as symptom diaries, some of which are free. It's important to choose the method that will work best for *you*, because getting accurate information for your health professional will help both of you find the best strategies for your illness. But please do not become

Date: 8 Feb 2014 Wake time: 6.30 Sleep time: 10.30	Headache severity on a scale of 1 to 10 1 = very mild 10 = very severe	Other symptoms (e.g. nausea, vomiting, aura, yawning, etc.)	Medication use and any other intervention (e.g. lying down in darkened room)	Activities or events (e.g. work, social, weather, bowel movement, menstrual cycle)
6.00				Very close weather, cloudy but no rain
7.00		Yawning and nausea Smell of partner's aftershave really bothered me	Anti-sickness medication	
				Went out last night so was late to bed (but not by much, only about 23.30) and only had one glass of wine with food.
8.00	5	Yawning and nausea		
9.00	5	Yawning and needed to go to the loo (urine)		
10.00	5	Aura on left side of head	Ibuprofen	
11.00	8	Pain and aura on left side of head	Had to go to bed and close the curtains	5 days after last period Work ok, bit stressful with deadlines
12.00	8	Pain and aura on left side of head	In bed	
13.00	8	Pain and aura on left side of head	In bed	
14.00	7	Pain diminishing, aura still there	In bed 2nd dose of ibuprofen	
15.00	7	Pain diminishing, aura gone	In bed	
16.00	5	Just pain behind left eye	Out of bed	
17.00	3	Just pain behind left eye but less		
18.00				
19.00				
20.00				
21.00				
22.00				
23.00				

Figure 6 Completed daily symptom diary for migraine

overly worried or stressed about keeping a perfect diary; any and all additional details that the doctors have about your symptoms will help them to diagnose your condition. Do not make yourself more ill by trying to note down minute details of your symptoms! Finally, diary-keeping can also be a good way to track your progress and any fluctuations in your condition. Sometimes it's unbelievably hard to remember what you were like last week or last month, or even yesterday! Therefore, having a diary where you can see that you have improved over time, even if only a little at the beginning, can be very motivating and empowering.

Routines

For all the conditions in this book, a good routine is incredibly important. Although this may seem obvious, it is very easy to get out of a routine once you start to feel unwell and, at times, it can be difficult to stick to a regular pattern in life. This can be especially tricky if you have a family and other dependants such as elderly parents, or irregular working hours. If this is the case, then it is imperative that you discuss your condition with others and build up a social support network. If your nearest and dearest are finding it hard to understand your illness, there is advice for friends and family in Chapter 8. Chapter 8 contains hints and tips on how to explain your illness to your loved ones, work colleagues and friends. The most important aspects of a routine are:

- waking and going to bed at approximately the same time each day;
- eating regular meals, including healthy snacks to maintain energy levels;
- taking medication at the same time every day.

It is also important to add in some activities to make you feel better, such as relaxation or meditation, and things that you enjoy, such as hobbies. Relaxation or meditation exercises can be done in very brief periods, for instance just five or ten minutes at a time. These activities are vital because if you are at home feeling rotten, you need to find activities to distract yourself. Or start new hobbies that you can incorporate into your life even though you are ill. Hobbies such as reading, craftwork and even looking up your family tree (there are many websites for this nowadays and it is very popular!) can be carried out in short bursts, can be very fulfilling and can also be increased when you start to feel better. Illness intrusiveness (see Chapter 3) is detrimental because the illness intrudes into previously valued life domains and interests, so people need to find replacement or displacement activities.

Hence, if genealogy is of interest to you (and perhaps you don't know if it is but it might be exciting to find out), then you could start your search online. You may not even be able to sit at a computer desk at this point but perhaps you have a tablet or laptop that you could use in bed until you are well enough to sit at a desk. This and many other hobbies can be very absorbing but do not require a great deal of energy.

> Although I can't always do everything round the house that I want to, like all the washing and cleaning, I've found that cooking – well, baking, really – takes me to a different place. I guess it's 'cause you have to concentrate to get the amounts right, so it takes my mind off the aches and pains. Of course I can't stand the whole time like I did so I have a stool in the kitchen now and then, and that seems to work rather well.
>
> (BR, with FMS)

If there's a party or special occasion that you want to go to, it is also good to go to the event, otherwise life may be rather beige! If you go out, it may just be important to make sure that you make it as comfortable for yourself as possible by working out the best route for getting there (this may mean making fewer changes on the train or ensuring that you have a lift with someone who is aware of your condition), perhaps booking into a hotel very near to the venue so that you can go back and take time out (in general, most people probably do this as intense social occasions like weddings can be rather overwhelming!) and checking ahead that the accommodation is quiet – for example, not above the bar! Hence, going to a big social event may take a bit of planning but it is important to maintain the fun things in life even though they may disrupt the routine in the short term.

Diet

A good, balanced diet is beneficial to everyone, not just people with an invisible illness. However, this can be difficult to maintain if you're feeling very unwell and completely lacking in energy, as a great many do with conditions such as IBS, FMS and CFS/ME. Keeping well hydrated is a good start to maintaining the body's physiological balance. Two litres of water a day (roughly eight glasses) is the general guidance. This may seem a lot at first, but in time it will become the norm. Limiting caffeinated drinks such as tea, coffee and cola will help to keep the body hydrated, because these beverages are diuretic. If short-term memory is a problem, simply keep a tally on a notepad or on a smartphone; indeed, reminders can also be set on a phone to take a drink! Again, this is 'general' good advice, so don't worry if one day you forget to drink the entire two litres, it is simply a beneficial habit to form because migraines and fatigue can be worsened by dehydration.

Migraines, fatigue and sensitivities to the environment can also be heightened by erratic changes in blood sugar levels. Foods high in sugar and very processed foods, such as cakes, biscuits, white bread and fizzy drinks, can cause sugar levels to spike and then drop dramatically. People with many of the disorders in this book appear to be sensitive to such changes, and so eating food high in protein and slow-release carbohydrates, such as non-starchy vegetables (spinach, kale, tomatoes, broccoli, cauliflower, cucumber, onions and asparagus), sweet potatoes, nuts and quinoa can help to maintain even blood sugar levels. Of course, being 'good' all the time can become a bit miserable so the occasional favourite naughty treat (say double chocolate fudge cake!) is of course fine.

Sleep hygiene

As discussed in Chapter 4, sleep is very important in invisible illnesses. Of course, it's important for everyone but perhaps more vital for people with long-term conditions to get good-quality sleep. There are some simple steps that you can take to help you to sleep better. With practice, these can become part of your normal routine and can help you regulate your sleep. However, it must be pointed out that in long-term fatiguing conditions such as CFS/ME, sleep can be very disrupted and so you may need additional help in the form of psychological and pharmacological aids (see Chapter 6). Here is some advice on what constitutes 'good' sleep hygiene:

- In addition to limiting the amount of tea, coffee and other caffeinated drinks (or drinking decaffeinated tea, coffee and colas instead, especially after lunchtime), it is also beneficial to steer clear of alcohol before bedtime. This may seem counter-intuitive because alcohol can make you sleepy (thus helping sleep onset), but it actually disrupts later stages of sleep as the body tries to metabolize the alcohol, resulting in arousal or wakefulness.
- If you like your main meal in the evening, try to have this earlier rather than later in the evening. In general, high-protein foods (such as meat, fish and eggs) are best at lunchtime, whereas carbohydrate-rich foods (such as pasta, bread and potatoes) are good in the evenings because these can make you feel sleepy. Chocolate also contains caffeine so it is probably a good idea to pass on a slice of fudge cake at bedtime.
- Exercise can help not only with symptoms but also with sleep

quality. Exercises like yoga can be particularly good in the evening to help the mind and body relax before bed.

- Hot baths just before bed may help also, as it's good for the body to start off hot in bed and then gradually cool down, rather than be cold and need time and energy to warm up.
- Rumination (see Chapter 4) can affect sleep. You might find yourself going over and over your current problems, things that have happened in the past, or things that might happen in the future. Techniques you can use to stop ruminating are discussed below, but if you feel you need additional support, your GP should be able to refer you for a course of talking therapy.
- It is best to limit the amount of stimulating equipment in the bedroom. This means that televisions, computers, smartphones and video games should be cleared from the bedroom. If you find a TV programme helps you fall asleep, try to watch it in the living room, then move to the bedroom when sleepy. It helps to get ready for bed, for example brushing your teeth, before sitting down to watch TV so that you can go straight to sleep afterwards without having to do an activity. But it's not a good idea to watch anything too exciting as this will stimulate the mind – think David Attenborough rather than David Beckham!
- Try to avoid naps in the daytime. (This may not be possible if you have CFS/ME.)
- Make your bedroom as comfortable as possible with gentle lighting and a temperature that suits you. If you live in a quiet area, it can be beneficial to leave a window open at night to ensure that there is enough fresh air.
- If you don't live somewhere quiet, a fan can help with keeping the air moving and also it will block out some external noise. There are also many different kinds of noise machines that can help to block out unwanted sounds. They produce a range of sounds, from white noise (which sounds like the static on a TV) to more natural sounds such as rainfall, ocean waves and heart beats. It may seem strange to think of adding more noise to your environment but the key here is that these sounds are steady and regular, rather than abrupt and startling, so they can help you to drift off and stay asleep.
- For disorders other than Ménière's disease and MdDS, earplugs can help to shield you from night-time noise. Inexpensive earplugs can be bought at any chemist and are usually made of foam or silicone. They may be disposable or longer-lasting. Larger high-street chemists also often have hearing care departments that can custom-make earplugs if you are very sensitive to noise. These can be quite expensive but should last many years.

- Natural light is very important for the sleep–wake cycle, and this can be something that is very hard for people with long-term illnesses to get enough of. If you are too unwell to go for a walk, try to sit outside if possible. (This will also help you to acquire vitamin D, which has been shown to be low in some illnesses and also in the general population in less sunny countries like the UK.) Light boxes can also help, but natural, outdoor light is best.
- Waking up naturally with daylight can also help the sleep–wake cycle. This of course can be very difficult in the winter when the days are very short, but there are a number of light alarms on the market these days that gradually fill the room with light, reproducing the sun coming up in the morning. These clocks also do the opposite at night-time, with light gradually diminishing to help the body gently fall asleep.
- Relaxation exercises can also help us to fall, and stay, asleep. A couple of simple techniques are outlined later in this chapter.

Sleep restriction

If your sleep pattern has become particularly bad and the general sleep hygiene guidance does not help, you may want to try a technique called sleep restriction. Our bodies follow a 24-hour cycle called the circadian rhythm (see Chapter 4). Through illness and other things (shift work, stimulating substances such as caffeine, and stress) this natural rhythm can become disturbed. By using sleep restriction, you may be able to 'reset' your body clock. But do note that this technique should not be used indefinitely; rather sleep restriction should be viewed as a tool when sleeping patterns have become very erratic.

To use this technique, first you need to calculate how well you sleep at this point in time, known as sleep efficiency. To do this, divide the time you are actually asleep by the time you are in bed, then multiply this by 100, which will result in a percentage – (time asleep ÷ time in bed) × 100. When calculating sleep efficiency, include only time in bed at night not any time in bed during the day. In general, healthy people have about 90 per cent sleep efficiency. On the opposite end of the scale, insomniacs may have only 5 per cent sleep efficiency.

Here is an example of a sleep efficiency calculation: say that you are in bed for eight hours but sleep for only six. The calculation would be: (6 ÷ 8) × 100 = 75, meaning that your sleep efficiency is currently 75 per cent. Do this every morning for two weeks so that you can ascertain an average sleep efficiency. You may want to use a sleep app on your smartphone to show you how much time you have slept, but bear in mind that these won't work if you have a memory foam mattress, because a memory foam mattress doesn't move as much as a regular one as you sink into it. Apps use movement to detect wakefulness. Sleep trackers that come as part of more general activity trackers are easier to use and can calculate sleep efficiency for you, but these come at a cost. Of course you can simply write down the estimations of time in bed and time asleep if this is more suitable for you.

Before you start restricting your sleep, it is important to rise at approximately the same time each day. To do this, set your alarm clock to wake you at a time you think is in tune with your body every day for one week. The time you naturally wake up is different for everyone so don't feel obliged to wake up at 8 a.m. just because your partner does, while you are attempting sleep restriction. By getting up at the same time each day, your body will become accustomed to this pattern. This is key when conducting sleep restriction so that you can accurately increase your sleep time in bed.

However, to begin sleep restriction, you must limit the time you spend in bed to the actual number of hours you sleep. Going back to the example above, even if you spend eight hours in bed on average but have found that you sleep for only six of these hours, then the sleep restriction programme starts with a six-hour period in bed. To do this, work back from your regular waking time. For instance, if you normally wake up at 9 a.m., then you need to go to bed at 3 a.m. This may seem quite shocking and an odd way to help with sleep problems but it has been shown to be effective. You will need to be disciplined in this first stage of sleep restriction, as it may feel unnatural. Indeed, you may feel even worse initially but do stick with it. However, if you simply find these timings too difficult, you can alter the time you go to bed and wake up (for example, by setting a wake time of 6 a.m. and going to bed at midnight). After all, you know your body best and what it's capable of.

When you wake up in the morning, calculate your sleep efficiency once again. You may notice that your sleep efficiency has risen slightly and this is the purpose of sleep restriction. For the remainder of the week keep to this schedule unless you find that your sleep efficiency has not improved. If this is the case, reduce the amount of time again to the time you are actually asleep. However, if you find that you are sleeping for the full six hours, at the end of the week increase your time in bed to six hours and 15 minutes. Therefore, now you will be going to bed at 2.45 a.m. instead of 3 a.m. You can use bigger increments such as 30 minutes but do remember that this is a gradual process so avoid making large leaps in terms of time in bed because this will limit the effectiveness of the technique.

After you find that you are sleeping for six hours and 15 minutes for a couple of weeks, you can increase the time you spend in bed even more. During this process you should continually calculate your sleep efficiency to ensure that it is not getting worse again. Figuring out what level of sleep efficiency is reasonable for you is your decision. If you have an illness, such as CFS/ME, in which sleep disturbance is a known problem, aiming at 90 per cent sleep efficiency may be overly ambitious. Aiming at 75–85 per cent may be a more achievable goal.

A programme of sleep restriction should ideally be carried out slowly and gently over about six weeks. Hopefully at this point you will be sleeping for most of the time you spend in bed. In addition, your day-time sleepiness should have decreased, and other symptoms, such as cognitive function and mood, may also have improved.

Pacing

Related to routine is the practice of pacing. Pacing is similar to GET (see Chapter 6) in the sense that a baseline level of activity is gauged first. However, it differs in that the aim is not to use all your energy to get tasks done but rather to balance activities with rest periods. This technique may help people to maximize the amount they can do by breaking activities down into categories, such as social, mental and physical activities. An activity log can help with figuring out which kind of tasks produce symptoms, and this information can then be fed into the decision-making process about what type of activity to do in a set time period, how long to do it for and what time of the day to do it. Pacing can be helpful for all the illnesses in this book, as most people with long-term conditions experience fatigue or pain.

> I was housebound for a year, and for a lot of that time I was bed-bound. At that time I felt that everything was chaotic – my sleeping patterns were all over the place, I couldn't walk unaided and I spent most of the day either in bed or sitting in a chair, as everything I did tired me out so much. A colleague who I had worked with phoned me, and offered to send me materials about CFS/ME. Some of this was about pacing and routine. I decided to make a rough timetable of activities for myself. So I would schedule in a time to get up, followed by, say, ten minutes of meditation, followed by a short walk (sometimes just from the bedroom to the lounge), followed by listening to the radio or phoning someone. So that I paced myself within each day. At first my activities were limited to five or ten minutes and in between, a rest of between 10 and 30 minutes. I did the activities whether or not I felt like doing them and rested even if I didn't think I needed a rest. Sometimes the activity was

simply reading a page of a book. As I became a bit better, the walks got longer (walking round the garden) but I still scheduled proper rests throughout the day – either in bed or in an armchair. I was very strict with myself, and I think it helped me, my life was very restricted, but was no longer chaotic, and I found that very helpful.

(CW, with CFS/ME)

Exercise

Exercise can be very difficult with an invisible illness, but gentle exercise can help some people with their symptoms. You may be thinking that this is a ridiculous idea because your symptoms are so bad that exercise is impossible – this is why it is extremely important to seek advice on appropriate exercise rather than try to force yourself to do the types of exercise that you may have been able to accomplish before the onset of illness. For some fatiguing conditions, such as CFS/ME, a particular form of therapy, GET, may be appropriate (see Chapter 6), and for other illnesses associated with pain, such as FMS, it is best to see an occupational therapist or physiotherapist, who can create a tailored programme for you as an individual and your symptoms and function.

Exercises for balance problems

For people with Ménière's disease or MdDS (or anyone who has problems with balance) special techniques known as vestibular exercises can help. These exercises use head movements that can actually cause dizziness, but it is important to carry on with the techniques because, as with any other form of exercise, tolerance can be built over time. The idea is to use the activities that cause symptoms in a controlled and purposeful way, starting off with small periods of time and then building up so that eventually symptoms are not produced during movement. This should also help you to regain confidence in daily activities so that you can go about your day-to-day life without the fear of dizziness and imbalance.

Here we outline a few examples. Please note that when you first try these exercises, you should have another person in the room with you in case your symptoms flare up and you need help to steady yourself. Persistence is key here, and these exercises should be carried out at least three times a day for between 6 and 12 weeks or until the dizziness stops completely. This is important because quitting before the dizziness is totally resolved increases the likelihood of a relapse. To gauge this, feelings of dizziness should be gone for a period of two weeks before the exercises are stopped for good. (They of course can always be restarted if symptoms return.)

1 Sit down comfortably in a chair and begin by bending your head down to look at the floor, then gradually up to look at the ceiling, ensuring that you lead your head with your eyes, which should focus first on the floor and then the ceiling. This exercise should be repeated ten times. Then, stop, take a break and wait for any dizziness to go away. After 30 seconds repeat the entire process twice more.
2 Again while sitting, start by turning your head to the right and then to the left, leading your head again with your eyes. (Think of it like watching the ball in a tennis match.) Then turn your head at a speed fast enough to cause dizziness but not so fast that you strain your neck. Go back and forth ten times, and then wait for 30 seconds or until the dizziness stops. Then the whole process should be repeated twice more.
3 Simply change from a sitting to a standing position and then back again 20 times. To make this more difficult, do the exercise with your eyes closed.
4 While standing up, throw a small ball from one hand to another, just above eye level. To move to the next level, throw the ball under one knee.
5 With assistance – as this one is a bit harder – stand with your heels together and look forward, holding your balance.
6 Again with assistance, stand on one foot and hold your balance, then try to do it with your eyes closed.

This is not a full list of vestibular exercises but it is hoped that from these examples it is clear that the techniques can easily be tried and practised at home (some with a partner at hand). By doing these exercises regularly, it is possible to retrain your brain to interpret information in a way that doesn't bring on symptoms. By creating the very symptoms that you wish to bring to an end, symptoms can be prevented as the brain comes to tolerate and interpret more accurately the information from the vestibular (balance) system.

Techniques to help stop rumination

Although we have mentioned the term 'rumination' several times in this book, it may be useful to define exactly what this word means. Rumination is a type of repetitive thought that is negative – not just the fleeting gloomy thought that may fly through your head but rather a continuous, downbeat monologue running repeatedly in your mind without a break. Rumination and worrying are key characteristics of anxiety and depression and, although these are not the cause of your illness (see Chapter 4), it is not unusual to feel anxious and depressed when your body no longer feels as if it's your own and your life has been turned upside down. On the contrary, they are perfectly normal responses to long-term illness. Also, let's be honest here; we *all* ruminate at times, whether we have an illness or not. Perfectly healthy people ruminate and worry about things – these are very common thought processes. It is only a problem if the repetitive thoughts stop you from getting good-quality sleep and affect your life in other negative ways, such as having an impact on your relationships and preventing you from moving on in life.

Examples

There are many different repetitive thoughts that may cause us difficulty but there are several ways in which you can combat rumination. Here are some examples.

1 Constantly thinking about the worst things that can happen can be problematic because it can prevent us from moving forward in life. (Being overly optimistic can also be a problem too but this is much less common.) For instance, think about the hypothetical wedding that you want to go to and the things you may need to do to make it manageable, such as leaving the reception for an hour to have a rest. The very idea of doing this may fill you with dread because you may think that other people will view you as moody or a kill-joy. However, this is a prediction rather than an actual script of what will happen on the day. Ask yourself if this is really the most likely outcome. Wouldn't most people's focus be on the happy couple? Or even the food? It may be a bit of a blow to your ego but most people spend far more time thinking about themselves and their needs than anyone else. Isn't it more likely that others will simply accept that you have pottered off to freshen up and think nothing more of it? Next, think about a thought pattern that could occur when you come back to the wedding. Worrying what other people think about you and deciding it must be bad is called mind-reading (even though we know that it is impossible to read others' minds). Did you see the woman on your table give you a funny look and assume all at once it is because she thinks you are rude for leaving? This is an assumption; it is not based on evidence. The 'look' is not evidence because you are making an inference; she could simply be thinking, 'I wish I had done what that person did and take a break, I'm so tired of listening to people rabbit on!' Assuming that the wedding guest thinks you're a bad person for retreating from the celebrations is mind-reading, and if you start to feel that you are going through this process, ask yourself if these are actually

the other person's thoughts or yours. How do you know that other people think you are rude? Have they said this? If they asked how your rest was, could it be that they wished that they had thought to book a hotel close by so that they could do the same? Try to look for the more balanced view of the situation rather than focus on the most terrible interpretation. Remember, people mostly think about themselves, not you!

2 A type of repetitive thought that can often keep you awake at night is the 'should–must' way of thinking. When at the wedding 'should' you have spoken to the bride's father more? 'Must' you email the man who gave you his business card straightaway even if you're feeling the after-effects of going to the wedding? This way of thinking is all about expectations. Take a step back from yourself and ask if these expectations are realistic. The family would have appreciated your attendance regardless of how long you spoke to the bridal party (again, their focus would be on the day going smoothly and making sure the guests are happy, with probably very little attention paid to each individual). What this means is that the expectations are ones that you have set for yourself. It is useful to ask whether they are too high. Are they always impossible to reach? What would be more realistic expectations? Perhaps attending the wedding is sufficient to show you care (it most likely is). Do you need to send that email right away? Why? Even if you said you would, is it really such a big deal if you wait for a few days? Isn't the other guest likely to be travelling home and recovering too? Basically, this repetitive thinking is putting a great deal of pressure on you and it's important to give yourself a break. Most situations are not life-or-death and, even if they are, you will have done the best you could in the situation within your capacity. Be kind to yourself.

3 Similar to the above is the 'critical-self' rumination. Do you constantly beat yourself up and criticize every small detail of your life and things you've done? To break this pattern, ask yourself, 'What would people who really know me say about me?' Are you completely responsible for things that perhaps have not turned out brilliantly in the past? Or was it a combination of circumstances, some of which were beyond your control? Situations are rarely simple and can certainly be viewed from many angles – try to look for the less critical interpretations.

4 When you are unwell for a long time, it can be very difficult not to see the worst in all aspects of life. This 'mental filtering' can be altered, however. This is within your power even if some of your physical symptoms are not. Ask yourself if you are filtering out the positives. Also ask, 'Am I concentrating only on the bad stuff?'

and 'Is there a more balanced or realistic view?' If your condition is very severe, this may simply involve noticing that it is a pleasant day or that you are enjoying the book you are reading. Recovery can at times be slow and often incomplete, but it is beneficial to appraise the small steps rather than just the set-backs. Reading this book is a positive activity because you are actively trying to improve your health. While life can be incredibly difficult with a long-term illness, if we can see some rays of light, it will not only lift our mood but could also help our symptoms.

5 Black-and-white thinking can also cause us to ruminate. Situations are rarely all good or all bad, all right or all wrong, black or white. Do you find that you evaluate life in this way? Does it have to be 'all good' to be OK? Actively looking for the shades of grey can turn negative repetitive thoughts into more constructive ones. 'I may not be completely well but at least I know my diagnosis and can do things to help myself' is a more useful approach than 'I am not 100 per cent where I used to be, so what's the point in trying?'

6 If you go to the nth degree in your thoughts and the outcome is always terrible, then you may be catastrophizing – in other words, thinking that every situation will end badly. Going back to the hypothetical wedding reception, if you catastrophize about attending the event too much beforehand, it will be very hard actually to go! This type of thinking could be somewhere along the lines of, 'If I go, I'll have to stay up later than I would normally do, and this could make me severely ill again, so I shouldn't go,' or 'If I go and find it difficult to talk to people, I will lose friends and then be in a worse situation than I am now.' These may be possibilities, but they are unlikely. Yes, you may feel a bit rotten after the event but now you know about stress reduction, good sleep hygiene and the importance of exercise and routine, so you can get back into your patterns when you get home. Now that you understand more about your illness, it is possible to exert more control over it and your life. People may react negatively to you but this could be because they don't understand your illness (see Chapter 8). It is more likely that you will enjoy the event, even if you are a bit tired by the end, and that others will have been happy to see you.

In general, if you are having repetitive thoughts, ask yourself if they are helpful or unhelpful. If unhelpful, try to reappraise the situation in a more balanced, realistic way. It can also be very useful to set aside time each day to consider the problem that is causing repetitive thoughts – so, tell yourself that you will think about the problem at a particular time, say 9 p.m., and mull over your problems for

15 minutes and then tell yourself to stop. This technique can contain the rumination and prevent repetitive thoughts from constantly entering the mind. But the trick here is to do the thinking at the time set, otherwise your mind will continue bombarding you with thoughts throughout the day and night! Writing problems down at a set time can also be beneficial and this is a rather more concrete way to allocate thinking time.

Relaxation techniques

Relaxation is important for everyone but possibly more fundamental to health if you have a long-term condition. There are many thousands of relaxation CDs and DVDs on the market but you needn't invest in these because the techniques are very simple indeed. In fact, there are now many free smartphone applications that talk through, step by step, relaxation exercises so you needn't spend a great deal of money (or any money) on learning to relax more deeply. The following techniques can be used either during the day for general relaxation or at night to aid sleep. If you want to try either technique in the day, sit in a comfortable chair with your feet placed on the ground (do not cross your legs). If you'd like to do them at night to help you to fall asleep, get into your preferred sleep position – simply use the best position for you as there are no 'right' or 'wrong' ways to lie down in terms of these exercises. Both these techniques encourage you to bring your attention inwards and, by using the specific sequences, it is less likely that repetitive thoughts will enter your mind. Basically, your mind will be busy but in a good way.

Examples

The first technique is known as a body search.

- Start by breathing in through your nose and out through your mouth.
- With every breath out, focus on the exhalation and relax.
- Now, for the next two or three exhalations, focus on either the chair or bed, feeling how it's supporting your body, and relax.
- Next, let your mind and your attention wander through your body. This does not have to be in any set sequence and should not be rushed. You may want to start with your fingertips – notice any sensations there: perhaps you can feel the weight of the duvet on them.
- Now move through the body. If you started at the fingers, move

up the arm and into the chest. Again, notice any sensations – your heartbeat, any warmth or coolness, perhaps you have experienced some twitching or needling sensations, gurgling or bubbling in the stomach or gut.

- When you feel a sensation, even any tension or stillness, acknowledge the sensation for a moment before continuing your journey through your body.
- You may start to notice that the amount of sensations you are feeling seems to be decreasing after a few minutes, and this is normal.
- If you are doing this technique to help you to fall asleep, continue. If you are doing this for general relaxation, take the tour until you reach your toes, then allow yourself a few more breaths before gradually returning to the outside world.

Counting rhythmically with your breaths can also act as a relaxation exercise.

- As above, start by breathing in through your nose and out through your mouth.
- Every time you take a breath, focus on the exhalation and relax.
- Now, for the next two or three exhalations, focus on either the chair or bed, feeling how it's supporting your body, and relax.
- Continue to focus on your exhalations, but now count from one to ten with each exhalation.
- Then count backwards from ten to one, again one exhalation per count.
- If you are using this technique to help with sleep initiation, you can count backwards from 99 until you fall asleep. If using this exercise in the daytime, repeat the forward and backwards counting the number of times it suits you. This technique can be carried out even in a busy schedule as it need only take a few minutes.

Meditation and mindfulness

Meditation is much like the relaxation exercises above. In fact the techniques above could be defined as meditation, as this is an umbrella term for many methods that enhance a relaxed state of being. Originally, many hundreds of years ago, meditation was used to deepen spirituality, but nowadays it is more often practised to reduce stress and promote both physical and emotional well-being. The most commonly used types of meditation include the following:

- Guided meditation uses imagery and visualization so that you can visit places or events that you find relaxing. Senses are key in this type of meditation, and the guide or teacher will encourage imaginings of touch, smell, sounds and even tastes.
- Mantra and transcendental meditation involves silently repeating a word or phrase that is calming. Transcendental meditation differs from mantra meditation as it teaches you to focus solely on the word or phrase to the exclusion of all other thoughts and stimuli. If practised successfully, it is claimed that a complete state of stillness and consciousness can be found.
- Yoga uses a series of postures and stretches along with breathing techniques in order to increase balance, concentration and flexibility in addition to calming the mind.
- There are methods that stem from traditional Chinese medicine, for instance qi gong and tai chi, which both use slow physical movement in conjunction with deep breathing exercises.

Mindfulness is also a type of meditation that can alleviate rumination and worry. It can help to reduce stress, which can be an important factor in long-term conditions (see Chapter 4) so trying to limit stress and its effects can certainly help symptoms and also general quality of life. Although mindfulness takes a great deal of its framework from Buddhism, it is not religious – it draws on some techniques used by Buddhists but not the philosophy as such. Like meditation, mindfulness teaches you to 'be in the moment', which is something that we often miss in our modern, frantic lives. This is because we are often on auto-pilot, quite unaware of our moment-by-moment experience. But we are capable of being in the moment and paying sustained attention to our internal workings. This is achieved by systematically paying attention to things such as physical sensations and perceptions or even imagining scenarios. However, a key difference between mindfulness and ordinary symptom monitoring is that this attention and awareness should be without judgement or evaluation – in other words, you are simply being aware of the sensation without analysing it. This may sound rather odd at first and it can feel strange when you first start trying out mindfulness! Mindfulness certainly requires practice, as it is a gradual and progressive learning curve. When a state of mindfulness is achieved, it is believed that a deeper and more vivid sense of life can be gained as the active nature of mindfulness can replace the reactive unconsciousness – the fight or flight responses discussed in Chapters 2 and 4.

There is a specific type of mindfulness called mindfulness-based stress reduction (MBSR), which is a structured programme that usually consists of eight to ten weekly sessions. Each session generally lasts two and a half hours and is sometimes followed by a full-day course at the weekend, but this of course will depend on the nature of the illness that the programme is designed to treat, as some groups may find this schedule too intense. MBSR is a group programme rather than a one-to-one treatment with a therapist. The group size can vary from 10 to 40 people. As mentioned previously, mindfulness is a skill that needs to be developed – practice is important, so often there will be 'homework' assigned. These out-of-class tasks are typically meditation practice, mindfulness-based exercise such as yoga, and using MBSR in everyday, perhaps stressful, situations.

As with the study on acupuncture in FMS (see Chapter 6), MBSR has been investigated across a number of studies in a meta-analysis. However, the researchers who looked at MBSR didn't choose a single condition but looked at the results across many different illnesses. The researchers found 20 studies with a total of 1605 participants. MBSR was seen to be beneficial in terms of quality of life and general well-being and reduction in anxiety and depression. Improvements were also seen in levels of pain, physical impairment and other medical symptoms. However, these studies don't tell us *why* mindfulness helps in these conditions, so more research is needed to uncover the mechanisms at play here.

Peer support and self-help groups

Self-help groups may not be your cup of tea. Or rather they may not seem to be something that you would see yourself doing – sitting with a group of people talking about illness. However, many groups are not like this at all. Generally, self-help groups are positive meetings where people share the experience of illness as well as positive experiences that may have little to do with the common condition. But, in the main, it can be incredibly liberating to meet others who have been through what you may still be dealing with, such as extreme confusion regarding symptoms, a body that no longer feels like your own (and that you can trust), difficulties and disappointments with the medical profession, problems at work and the pervasive guilt that can come with not being able to do what you used to do for others.

> I was very reluctant to join a self-help group after I was first diagnosed. My doctor suggested it and my gut reaction was, 'God, no, why would I want to be stuck in a room with other people with this illness, all moaning to one another!' But in the end I decided to give it a go and I thought if it was horrible I could just never go back! I'm not going to

lie and say it was wonderful at first – it's not like we had anything else in common other than fibromyalgia. In fact, I was one of the youngest people in the group. But over time, I have picked up a lot of helpful tit-bits about fibro and the email group sends links to research and talks. I don't read all these or even go to the talks but it's just nice to know that things are moving on with the condition. If the only people I had contact with to talk to about it were my family and doctors, I would feel like nothing is happening and probably quite depressed! With the group, I can talk about a symptom and I know the others will know exactly what I mean. This has been very liberating, even if we have nothing else in common! But actually, we do, as people are people, at the end of the day.   (AG, with FMS)

Summary and conclusion

In this chapter we have looked at ways in which you can actively help yourself and your illness, starting with keeping a detailed diary so that you can help the doctors make the correct diagnosis, moving on to the importance of a routine, a good diet, quality sleep and exercise, to ways in which you can help reduce negative repetitive thoughts and stress. In the next chapter we outline some hints and tips for how best to communicate with your family, friends, doctor and colleagues about your condition and needs. The next chapter also includes a guide written for those in your support network so that they can offer you appropriate help and understanding.

8

Hints and tips on how to deal with doctors, family, friends and work, and a guide for how others can help you

In this chapter, we include quotes from people who have found ways to interact successfully with health-care professionals, family and friends. We give some tips for discussing your condition at work – practical ways to get the most out of your interactions with others so that they can offer you support.

We also include a section specifically written for your family, friends and colleagues. You may want to give this to them and let them read the guidance in their own time. However, you might prefer to take the ideas from this section and chat them through with your supporters. It can be difficult to communicate aspects of invisible illnesses when you have one yourself, so use this guide as a basis for discussion. That way, you will be able to share your experiences openly and build strong support networks.

Getting the best from your health-care practitioner

I spent a long time feeling so angry, hurt and disgusted with the way I'd been treated by various doctors, I actually started to develop a bit of a phobia when going to the doctor's surgery. If my appointment ran late and I saw someone go in before me when I thought I should be next, so much emotion would rise that I could feel my heart pumping in my chest. By the time I would get in the doctor's office, I would be so emotional that it's no wonder that the doctor probably thought I was suffering from some sort of psychiatric illness! So, I took it upon myself to change this pattern with my most recent doctor. When I met her for the second time, I told her about all my various health problems and symptoms but said the most important thing was for us to develop a trusting relationship. I said that I knew she couldn't wave a magic wand and make everything perfect but if we could try to systematically deal with one thing at a time, that would be a good start. I think she was relieved and now I feel like it's more of a collaboration – we are working together to make my health as good as it possibly can be. Some things I can do myself and some things I need her help with. So far, this has been one of the best things I have done for my condition.

(RM, with MdDS)

As shown by this quotation, it will be most beneficial for you to develop a collaborative relationship with your doctor or health-care practitioner. If you have had negative experiences with people such as doctors, nurses, psychologists and physiotherapists, this may seem like unrealistic advice. However, most health-care professionals do want to help, they might just not know how to. The conditions in this book are still far from clear in terms of their precise cause. Also, there are many common symptoms in invisible illnesses, so it can take time to reach the correct diagnosis. This can be a very challenging time for both you and your doctor. Doctors are trained to make diagnoses and provide treatment, so if they are presented with a complex and confusing case, it may be frustrating for them also. This of course is nothing compared to what you're going through with your condition, but if you can help your health-care practitioner, he or she will be able to help you in turn. Some key tips to working with your doctor follow.

- Don't expect a diagnosis in one appointment. It can take time and you may need to see a number of specialists to reach a diagnosis. This may be hard but be as patient as you can. Getting the correct diagnosis is more important than getting a quick diagnosis.
- If you think you know what condition you have, ask your practice if any of the GPs have a specialist interest in that area and consult with that person if possible. Likewise, if you are referred to a specialist, for instance a neurologist for suspected migraine, request to be referred to one that has a migraine and headache clinic. You can often find doctors' specialist interests by searching on the internet.
- Give your health-care professional sufficient information to help with not only diagnosis but also treatment. This is where symptom diaries can really help (see Chapter 7).
- If you are starting a new treatment, keep a symptom diary because this will allow you to see more objectively if the therapy is helping. It is also helpful to note any side effects so these can be discussed with your doctor.
- In many invisible illnesses, different treatments work for different people, so you may have to try a few therapies to find the right one for you. It may be that a combination of techniques will help you

on the road to recovery, not just a single pill or treatment. Therefore, try to keep an open mind when discussing possible treatment
approaches with your health-care professional.

- Don't wait to start some of the self-help techniques while in the
  process of finding a diagnosis. Regular routines, a healthy diet and
  good-quality sleep are vital not only for people with invisible illnesses but for everyone throughout life.
- Remember that you have an active role to play in your recovery;
  don't expect your doctor to 'fix you' if there are also areas of your
  life that you could be addressing as well (for instance diet, stress or
  rumination).

Communicating with your family

Because they can't see the pain, they just didn't believe me for ages. My
mother-in-law told me many times to 'just snap out of it' and she said,
'If I were you I would be out and about enjoying my life, not sitting on
the sofa waiting for life to come to me!' This, as you can imagine, didn't
help me very much! It took me ages to stop just reacting to her stupid-
ity and explain fibromyalgia to her. It wasn't easy as she's a stubborn
woman, but with the help of some research papers from the internet
and books, and also her seeing me do things to help myself, she has
finally stopped berating me and is, at times, supportive. She can still be
a *****, however!   (BD, with FMS)

It can be incredibly upsetting to have close family members question
the existence of your illness. It can be very challenging for people
who have always been in good health to empathize and support a
relative who 'looks fine'. You may not feel that it's worth your while
to try and persuade your family member that you are 'really ill'
(and it may not be!), but bear in mind that building strong support
networks can help you in all areas of life, not just with your health.
If you choose to engage with any dismissive relatives, here are some
tips.

- Although you may be justified in feeling angry with their lack of
  support, try not to lash out at your family. They may feel just as
  confused and frustrated as you (though admittedly they are not
  experiencing the symptoms of an invisible illness), so reacting
  defensively will not help the situation.
- Accept that your family love you and may be struggling with
  seeing you unwell. This does not mean you should try to hide your
  symptoms from your family, but rather talk openly about your

condition and also the strategies you are using to deal with them.

- Some people simply don't know how to help. Tell them. This may be in a practical way like helping with housework or children, or in an emotional way by simply listening. Different people are better at different types of support, so bear this in mind. It may not be the best idea to ask your macho brother to be a shoulder to cry on or your elderly aunt to pick up the kids from school, so be realistic in your expectations.

- On the topic of realistic expectations, try not to expect one single person to provide all the support you may need. This is sage advice for everyone, at all stages of life. Relying too much, for example, on your spouse or partner can put undue pressure on him or her, which may, in turn, damage your relationship. We all need a number of people, not only family but friends, acquaintances and colleagues, to meet our needs.

- Show your family member the Guide for family, friends and colleagues on how to best support you, later in this chapter.

Maintaining friendships

At first I tried to go out all the time like always but eventually it just became too hard. I would get a severe migraine the next day which would last for three days. I guess even then I knew things like booze and coffee were triggers but I just didn't want to admit it. You feel like a freak if you have to not drink on a night out. It's also kinda boring – it's funny actually how boring my friends are when drunk! I guess when you're drunk too you just don't notice! I do a few things now – I try to do things like dinner and cinema rather than just the pub. This way I can drink a bit as it's with food. So I suppose it [the migraines] has changed me a bit in relation to friends. The good ones are totally happy to do dinner instead of drinking and I guess I don't see the rubbish ones that much anymore. But I actually think that would have happened anyway with getting older!   (PT, with migraine)

As with family, friends can often feel helpless when someone they care about is ill, can't do the activities they used to do and appears to be disengaging from social life. In the first instance, being honest with your friends is the best route to take. You may find that some are wholly supportive, while others are apparently dismissive of your condition. You may even find that some of your friends have invisible illnesses that you never knew about! Over time, good friends may seem to fall by the wayside. Again, as with relatives, this may be simply because they do not know how to support you, so do tell people how they can best be your friend. You should show friends the Guide for family, friends and colleagues on how to best support you later in this chapter. In addition, some tips for maintaining friendships when you have an invisible illness follow here.

- Suggest new activities or ways to communicate if you are struggling with old ones. For instance, like PT in the quotation above, instead of going to the pub suggest you meet over dinner. If you used to go to a high-impact exercise class but need to give your body a break from it, mention to your gym buddy that you'd like to try the yoga class for a while instead. If you have a friend who constantly texts you throughout the day, tell your friend that it would be nicer to hear his or her voice and have a phone call at a time when you feel good, whatever time of day this may be.
- As with family, give your friends some practical ways in which they can help you. Some people may simply not know what to do and because of this may keep their distance. If you give friends clear guidance, they will be in the best position to support you
- This may be an opportunity to rebalance some friendships. If you feel as if you are always the 'giver' in a particular relationship, be honest with your friend and say you need some support from him or her. Your friend may react badly to this but remember that you must put yourself first to recover the best possible level of health.
- Don't feel ashamed that you are now not as good a friend as you feel you should be. Life and relationships are full of ups and downs, and that's what friends are for!

Dealing with work

I discussed my diagnosis of CFS/ME with my line manager first, at which point I explained the illness and its symptoms. He was very supportive about my condition and said the company would do whatever they could to support me. He discussed it with human resources and they advised me to try working from home one day a week and to monitor the effectiveness of this. Although this did help, my symptoms did not improve so, two months later, I had a further conversation with my boss and HR. At this point, they arranged for me to speak to an occupational health adviser. I explained my symptoms to the OH therapist, who then wrote up and sent her advice to my line manager and HR. She advised reducing my hours/days and facilitating regular rest breaks, as well as avoidance of rush-hour travel. Due to work pressures, I was unable to follow this advice and my health deteriorated to the point where I was unable to continue working and was advised by my GP to take a com-

plete break for one month. The company supported me in doing this
and we will be discussing my return to work imminently.
(SE, with CFS/ME)

Most workplaces have policies to deal with ill health and sick leave.
It's advantageous to know the details of these so ask your HR manager
for the organisation's policy document. However, if you are unwell the
first point of contact is generally your line manager. Your line manager
may be able to arrange more flexible working conditions on his or
her own authority but this may need to be discussed with the HR
manager, as seen in the quotation above. At this point, or possibly
further down the line, you may be asked to visit the occupational
health (OH) department (if your organisation has one). This can feel
like a frightening and uncertain time so if you are a member of a
union, speak to your representative about this process. If you do not
have a union or are not a member, you can ask a colleague to support
you.

In the OH appointment, the assessor will ask you about your condition and evaluate if you are fit for work. You (or your representative
or advocate) may want to look at your organisation's fitness for work
policy before this session so that you are aware of the criteria that you
are being guided by. The assessor may suggest you take time off work,
work from home for a period or work part time. This will usually be
decided with your input and that of your line manager and HR manager. To help you through this process, some tips follow here.

- Make sure you have written documentation of all conversations
  and agreements with regard to your new working pattern. This is
  to ensure that you are not pressured to work more than has been
  approved in relation to your current health. Keep these documents
  safe and refer back to them if you begin to feel compelled to do
  more than was agreed.
- If you feel your line manager is unsupportive, speak directly to your
  HR department. Most organisations have policies against discrimination, including discrimination on the basis of invisible conditions. Speaking to the HR department may be a better option than
  going above your line manager's head by speaking to his or her
  manager. The aim is to go back to work, so avoiding any unnecessary frictions can only be a good thing.
- Make sure you provide any documentation from your doctor that
  is requested. However, this should be reasonable and in relation to
  your current illness (so not your complete medical notes).
- Re-evaluate your health. You may need a chunk of time off work

to rest, see specialists and reduce stress, but your needs will change over time. Keep in touch with your HR and occupational health departments, as it may take a few alterations in working patterns to find the one that suits you.

- Generally, return to work is a phased approach, so bear this mind. It is unlikely that you will be asked to take on board all the tasks that you used to have responsibility for immediately after returning to work. If this seems to be the case, discuss returning workload with your manager, as a phased approach is advised. If you feel under pressure to do more work than has been agreed, be as assertive as you can be with your line manager or discuss this with your union or a trusted colleague.

- If at any point you feel that you have been treated unfairly in relation to either the occupational assessment or workload when returning to your job, seek help and advice either from your union or from a legal representative (for instance, at the Citizen's Advice Bureau, which is free and confidential).

- Finally, you may find that you do not wish to return to your previous career. Your health may have highlighted something important, for instance, that your life has been too demanding and unsustainable. Take time (if you can within your financial situation) to consider your working desires. You may find that you'd like to retrain in a completely different discipline. Alternatively, you may view work differently now, perhaps as being less important than you once believed it was. We all need money to survive so you may feel that you have no option but to go back to work. If so, explore carefully whether there are things you can do to make your working life more enjoyable and sustainable. Perhaps you often took on more work than others because you like to help people. If this is the case, you may need to change your behaviour at work and protect your time more carefully.

Guide for family, friends and colleagues on how to best support you

This section has been written directly for those in your support network so the characters in the examples rotate between family members, friends and workmates. This is to demonstrate the ways in which simple changes in interactions can help both you and those in your close circle to maintain good and valuable relationships. In addition, there is advice on ways for these people to support you in a practical sense. Therefore, please bear in mind the tips are aimed at those that surround you and are voiced in that sense.

Support tip 1: Acknowledgement

It may have been difficult for whoever has given you this guide to do so. Having an invisible illness can be incredibly disorientating and can also elicit feelings of guilt, shame and 'not being good enough'. Therefore, it may have been hard for your friend to admit to you that he has an illness and needs your support and understanding. By letting others know about the illness, your friend has taken an important step in improving his health. You may feel that it's appropriate to acknowledge this explicitly to your friend. However, simply by saying you will do what you can to be there for him is enough and shows that you're willing and able to offer support.

Support tip 2: Try not to give advice

This may seem counter-intuitive but it is unlikely your relative wants to hear about what your best friend's aunty's neighbour has done to 'cure' herself of FMS (or any other condition for that matter!). Because numerous invisible illnesses don't have a clear cause, many people try various treatments and therapies to rid themselves of symptoms. While your advice will undoubtedly stem from a good place (you want to help your relative), the reality is that she could:

- be overwhelmed by all the advice well-meaning people are giving;
- feel guilty that your best friend's aunty's neighbour has been 'cured' but she hasn't been, and therefore blame herself;
- simply want you to listen, not offer suggestions.

Support tip 3: Don't ask people how they're doing if you don't want to hear the truth

Being able to listen is one of the best types of support you can offer your colleague. But you must be prepared really to listen. This is quite different from the day-to-day 'How are you?' with the general reply 'I'm fine, thanks, and you?' Your colleague may be feeling like utter rubbish and could be struggling with symptoms. People with long-term conditions often find that others are sympathetic for a time but that after a while the rivers of sympathy run dry. They notice that people's eyes start glaze over when being told that today is not a great day (again). If you don't feel that you can listen to a negative response to the 'How are you?' question, it may be better not to ask. However, what is much more valuable to your colleague is to listen. Don't feel under any pressure to try to 'fix' his situation and do not feel guilty that you can't. Simply be an open ear, as this type of support is priceless.

Support tip 4: Remember, invisible illnesses are invisible!

Even if your friend looks well, she may not feel well. This is one of the cruel features of invisible illnesses. It's not simply that people with conditions like CFS/ME may not look terrible, they may actually look very good. This is because no one wants to look ill or bad, so your friend may have made a great deal of effort to hide any outward signs (for instance, by wearing make-up to hide a pale complexion or by resting to ensure that she has enough energy to enjoy your meeting). Conversely, your friend may actually be having a rather good day with few symptoms. However, try not to assume that this means she is 'better' now, as most invisible illness fluctuate. Jumping to the assumption that 'because you look fine, you must be fine' will only make it more difficult for your friend to feel supported by you. Looks can be deceptive.

Support tip 5: Try not to be frustrated by cancellations

People with invisible illnesses will still *want* to do all the things they used to do before they became unwell, but they may not be able to. Especially at the start of his illness, your brother may continue planning nights out, weekends away and so on, and only near the time realize that he cannot make it because of symptoms or concerns about possible symptoms. Try not to get annoyed at this – your brother will not be cancelling without due cause, it is simply the reality of an unpredictable illness. But there are strategies you can use to help your brother to schedule events in a way that make them least likely to be cancelled at the last minute. While he's still getting to grips with his IBS, it may ease your brother's mind to know that there is a toilet available when travelling. For instance, taking a train which has numerous toilets on board may be a better option for a weekend away than booking a coach that usually only has one toilet, sometimes none.

Support tip 6: Keep in touch

It may feel at times that your workmate is pushing you away by cancelling arrangements, not returning your calls and apparently falling off the face of the planet, but she's not doing this intentionally. She will be feeling terribly guilty (even though she shouldn't) for not keeping in contact as much as she used to. If your friend is prioritising her health by limiting social activity, try to be supportive of this. Ask your colleague which method of contact is easiest for her. Email or text may be the best way to keep in contact because she can reply when she feels up to it. However, it is still nice to be asked to attend some events so don't stop all the invitations, just bear in mind that a hard-rock concert might not be the best outing for someone with Ménière's disease.

Support tip 7: Give practical support

Although listening to your friend and acknowledging her illness are very important in terms of the support you can offer, practical help is also invaluable. If your friend has children, you could suggest that you drop them off or pick them up from school. This would not necessarily need to be every day but even once a week may afford a degree of respite to your friend. Likewise, you could have your friend's children come to your house to play for a few hours at the weekend. For people without children, offering to help with housework, picking up medicines from the chemist, driving them to doctors' appointments and delivering food can all help enormously. It can be embarrassing for people to have to ask for practical support and your friend may have been struggling to keep up with daily life for some time. These apparently simple things can make a great deal of difference to the life of someone with an invisible illness.

Support tip 8: Don't imply that an illness is 'all in the mind'

By telling your cousin that his condition is 'all in his head' you are insulting him. You may have read other chapters of this book and seen that people with invisible illnesses can also have depression and anxiety. This does not mean that your cousin's symptoms are due to his low mood or bad outlook on life. In fact, it is the other way around – having an invisible illness can often create depression and anxiety because few people are likely to understand what he's going through. In addition, it can take time to receive a diagnosis. This period of uncertainty can be very stressful indeed, and we know that stress has a *physiological* impact on the body. By dismissing your cousin's illness as 'all in the mind', you will be adding to this stress and his sense of self-blame. Your cousin is not to blame for his illness and he is actively trying to help himself recover by reading this book. So do try to appreciate that while depression and anxiety can be features of an invisible illness (indeed of any illness), this does not mean that your cousin is 'mad' or 'crazy'.

Support tip 9: Help to reduce stress

As just mentioned, stress has a compounding effect when someone is unwell. By this we mean that stress will make your friend's health worse, just as continual stress will have an impact on your health. By following these tips you will already be supporting your friend and lowering her stress levels but you can also do some practical things. For instance, your friend may be trying to apply for financial assistance from the government. This can certainly be a stressful experience so offer to help your friend fill out the forms and collect information. If she has to go to an appeal, you may want to act as her advocate. There is a great deal of information on-line about the welfare and benefits processes but it can be exhausting to navigate. You can unburden your friend of this by doing some of the background research, ringing the welfare offices on her behalf and keeping notes of any advice she has been given. With many invisible illnesses, stress can lead to poor sleep quality, which again worsens symptoms. By helping your friend tackle some of the stressful situations she encounters, you will not only be helping her directly with that situation, but also limiting any worsening of her condition.

Support tip 10: Don't assume that being off work or home is an easy option

Your colleague has downgraded his workload to part time and started working from home. This is unlikely to have been by choice, and for some people this would have been a heart-breaking decision. However, another co-worker has made the following comment to you: 'Jim is so lucky, isn't he? Being able to "work" from home, watch television in his underpants and drink tea all day! That's the life!' While you may agree that having the odd day working from home can be pleasant for people in good health, you know that for those with an invisible illness it is more likely to have been a forced choice. You know your close colleague would have been given the option to work from home *only* if his symptoms were severe enough to justify this. Therefore, the comment from your other co-worker offends you, but you might not know whether to challenge it or stay silent and simply nod your head. Challenging people's misguided beliefs can be hard and you might not want to rock the boat at work. However, these beliefs lead to stigma, and research has shown us how damaging stigma can be to many groups, not just to people with invisible illnesses. (Just think of any minority group.) Therefore, we advise that you should strongly challenge this comment so that it doesn't run riot in your workplace and create an uncomfortable atmosphere for your close colleague when he returns to work. You could say something like, 'I really doubt that Jim is sitting in his pants playing the X-box while we are here working our socks off. I think it's more likely that he will be doing his best to keep his job in difficult circumstances. His pay may have been cut, which will undoubtedly be putting a strain on his finances and home life. So I think the last thing he needs is for us to be gossiping about him.' This way, you can nip any rumours in the bud, which is an incredibly worthwhile means of supporting your colleague and friend.

Final thought for supporting your relative, friend or colleague

If you are a relative, friend or colleague of someone with an invisible illness, we hope that you've found this guidance helpful. There are a great many misconceptions about people with these conditions and so the best possible support you can give is to tackle these mistruths. However, don't worry about having to say or do the perfect thing because, with all relationships, there are ups and downs and your friend will appreciate your efforts, even if at times he or she may not directly observe them.

Summary and conclusion

This chapter has been in two parts: one full of hints and tips for you to help communicate and get the best out of your support group, the other for your supporters to help them to offer you both emotional and practical care. In the next and final chapter we explore some interesting directions for research and treatments to show you that there are a great many researchers and scientists who have dedicated their careers to gaining a better understanding of invisible illnesses.

9

Future directions and conclusions

I've got MdDS, but it hasn't got me!   (JH, MdDS Foundation)

This final chapter explores some interesting research directions that may change the situation for people with invisible illnesses. Of course, research is a slow process and it does take time for the results of such studies to trickle down to health care, but it is important to see that there is progress and to know that there are scientists who are trying to untangle the complexity of such conditions and ultimately improve the lives of those with long-term illness.

From mice to men (and women!)

A lot of the time, research starts in the laboratory with animals, not humans, undergoing the testing. Although this may seem a world away from treatment, it is an important start and these studies, if successful, can then lead to trials with human participants. Over the past few years, groups of scientists have been investigating the guts of mice in an attempt to understand the link between gut microbiota and mentalistic phenomena such as emotions. The term 'microbiota' refers to the collections of micro-organisms that live in certain areas of our bodies, for instance, on the skin, in the mouth and in the gut. Each of these areas contains a different set of microbes (microbiota). A more common term for gut microbiota is 'flora' but this term isn't often used in scientific studies. The gut microbiota is made up of tens of trillions of micro-organisms, including over 1,000 known forms of bacteria. Every single person on the planet has an individual gut microbiota and, like fingerprints, no two are the same, although family members usually have more similarities than non-family members. However, about one-third of the micro-organisms in the gut microbiota are similar across the human race, so some interesting comparisons can be made.

The role of the microbiota is very important indeed for our health and well-being. This large body of micro-organisms that lives in the intestine (which can weigh up to two kilograms!) helps to digest food, produces some vital vitamins (B and K), acts as a barrier for the immune system and fights off other dangerous micro-organisms, helping to preserve the integrity of the intestinal mucosa. In addition to these fundamental roles, we are now beginning to understand that the gut microbiota is involved in brain development, pain thresholds and HPA axis responses (in Chapter 2 it was shown why the HPA axis could be involved in numerous long-term illnesses), and it was the initial studies in mice that illustrated this. This is because the gut has a signalling pathway to the brain, which is imperative for maintaining homoeostasis – the brain and the gut communicate in order for our internal environments to remain stable and healthy. Although the exact mechanisms of this brain–gut communication have been in question, recently some exciting findings have been emerging that have attempted to explain this communication in terms of gut microbiota.

Examples of such studies used 'germ-free' mice, which are rodents that are bred in conditions that exclude bacteria. This method allowed investigators to manipulate the gut microbiota in the mice and observe the effects. A number of different research groups have done this and introduced probiotics (i.e. 'good' bacteria) into the gut microbiota of the mice. These probiotics were found to moderate intestinal pain and sensitivity.

Of course, it is a large (and unscientific) jump to assume that the same effects would be found in human beings, so additional studies are being carried out to see if these findings can be upheld with human participants. One such study carried out by researchers at the School of Medicine in the University of California, Los Angeles (UCLA) recruited healthy women with no history of gastrointestinal or psychiatric illness and gave them a fermented milk drink that contained a range of probiotics. A comparison group was given a similar drink but without the 'good' bacteria. Then both groups were asked to consume the products for four weeks. The ground-breaking aspect of this study was not that the researchers simply asked the women how they felt after the four weeks elapsed and made comparisons, but rather that any differences between the two groups were observed directly via brain scans. The women who drank the probiotic products were shown to have decreased activity in areas of the brain that control the central processing of sensation and emotion, meaning that the women in the probiotic group were less sensitive to pain and better able to maintain a stable (good) mood.

This is a very encouraging finding when thinking about possible treatments for long-term conditions such as IBS and FMS. If probiotics do indeed influence the brain–gut pathway, then effective treatments may be developed to alter the gut microbiota, which, in turn, may offer effective symptom relief.

Diagnosis – using twenty-first-century technology

In addition to increasing our understanding of the mechanisms in invisible illnesses, a great deal of work is also concentrating on better and faster diagnosis. Professor Tony Buffington, from Ohio State University in the USA, believes that he and his team may have developed a quick and easy test for diagnosing FMS. Professor Buffington carried out a study that analysed blood samples with a high-tech, specialized microscope to see if differences could be detected in the samples of people with FMS, rheumatoid arthritis and osteoarthritis. The infrared microscope looked at the molecular pattern within the blood samples and the scientists were then able to differentiate accurately between these illnesses. As the blood samples needed for this type of analysis are only very small, they can be collected via a finger prick – only a few drops are required. This could have substantial implications in that a diagnostic test may be available in primary care, in other words at your local GP's surgery. FMS, like the other conditions in this book, is often difficult to diagnose, and people sometimes have to see numerous doctors over many years to be diagnosed. Lack of a diagnosis can cause a great deal of stigma, resulting in anxiety and depression, which is a very unjust state of affairs when someone is ill already. Therefore, this type of test has the potential to be 'game-changing' and to reduce the social and psychological impact of the condition.

There has also been some very encouraging work recently in the area of migraine diagnosis using structural brain scans, rather than functional scanning techniques. As you can imagine a lot of attention is being given to this brain scanning work for conditions where the cause is not clear, because it has the potential to show us what is happening differently in the brains of people with a long-term illness. A research group from the Departments of Neurology and Radiology at the University of Pennsylvania, again in the USA, with colleagues from the Department of Radiology of Tianjin, China, looked at the brain structure of three groups of people: those with migraine that included aura, those with migraine without aura, and healthy people (acting as a comparison group). This was quite a large study, with 170 people in total. The researchers were specifically interested in a part of the brain known as the circle of Willis, which is the system of arteries that is located at the base of the brain. This is an important cluster of blood vessels because it provides blood flow to the brain. The researchers found that an incomplete circle of Willis was more common in participants with migraine with aura than in the healthy participants. People that had migraine but without aura were also more likely to have an incomplete circle of Willis but this association was not statistically significant, which means that the researchers and others in the scientific community would need to carry out further work to decide if this is a consistent problem in people who have this type of migraine. Nevertheless, this finding could potentially be important as an explanation for migraine. Because the circle of Willis is key to blood flow in the brain, this incomplete structure may contribute to a decreased flow or less sustained flow. In other words the incomplete circle of Willis may produce a 'double-whammy' for people with migraine when coupled with another problem that has been found in those with migraine, that of neuronal hyper-excitability. Neuronal hyper-excitability is when a person's brain is over-active. This over-activity means that the brain needs more blood flow to function properly. If the blood cannot get to where it needs to be, unpleasant symptoms may arise, such as a migraine attack.

However, and even more crucially, this research may offer a more reliable way to diagnose migraine. If more studies are done using high-tech imaging and the same or similar results are found, there is the possibility that in the future instead of having to wait on average eight years for a diagnosis of migraine, a structural MRI (magnetic resonance imaging) scan may be all that is needed. However, it must be noted that even people without migraine can have an incomplete circle of Willis, so further work will be needed for this to constitute a clear diagnostic test.

Splitting, not lumping

In Chapter 2 we touched on the 'lump or split' debate – that is, whether scientists, researchers and medics should 'lump' a range of long-term conditions such as IBS, FMS and CFS/ME together as one 'functional somatic syndrome' or whether it would be better to spilt each condition up into more specific entities. Although there are still people who prefer the first approach, there are also researchers who are doing something known as phenotyping. A phenotype is a cluster of characteristics that can be observed and that develop in a person as a result of both genetics and the environment. You may have heard the 'nature or nurture' debate, which is the argument about whether certain characteristics or traits are inherited and so are due to our genes – nature – or whether they come about because of the life we have lived and our interaction with the outside world – nurture.

We now know that it is not as simple as one or the other but that genetic factors interact with environmental influences throughout the lifespan. However, we can still categorize or group people together in meaningful ways, and one study has looked at sleep as a way to define or 'split' the population of those with CFS/ME. Researchers based in the north of England and the Netherlands looked at the polysomnography of 343 people diagnosed with CFS/ME. Polysom-nography consists of measurements of brain activity, heart rate and respiration, and it is used to diagnose sleep disorders. Interestingly, the researchers found that over 30 per cent of the people with a diagnosis of CFS/ME in this study had a sleep disorder that could account for their symptoms. The remaining participants could be separated into four groups in terms of different types of sleep disturbance:

- people who found it difficult to fall asleep and had a smaller per-centage of both stage 2 and REM sleep;
- people who woke up more times each hour than the other groups;
- people who slept longer overall, had more REM sleep and woke up less during the night than the other groups;
- people who slept the least overall and woke up a lot even after ini-tially falling asleep.

This study demonstrated two very important points:

1 how essential it is for patients with long-term conditions to be diagnosed properly, because there are many treatments for sleep disorders;
2 by looking at phenotypes we can learn more about invisible illness and devise tailored treatments.

In fact, the next study by these researchers is going to do just that – give each phenotype a specifically created sleep-based treatment to test whether such treatments are effective. If these treatment programmes do prove to be useful in helping people with their symptoms, the current guidance for doctors could change.

Treatments that take into account the mind–body relationship

As well as more tailored or personalized treatments like the ones that are being developed from the 'splitting' or phenotyping studies, there is also starting to be a greater acceptance of the need for multifaceted approaches. This means that rather than long-term conditions being something that should just be treated with drugs or physiotherapy or psychological therapy, these illnesses should be attacked with combinations of treatments. A group of doctors and scientists from Brazil who have reviewed the results of a large body of scientific and medical research about FMS recently published a report in the journal *Current Pain and Headache Reports*. These experts concluded that a combined approach to the treatment of FMS is the best approach – that is, using both pharmacology and CBT in addition to encouraging exercise and other lifestyle changes. As it certainly appears that there is no single cause for the invisible illnesses that we have explored in this book, it makes sense that there will not be one single treatment. This greater acceptance of the complex nature of these disorders and also the importance of the interaction between the mind and body is a major shift in medicine and will, we hope, afford greater understanding and compassion as well as better treatments. Additionally, the insistence that invisible illnesses should be viewed as 'true' illnesses in the medical community will, in time, trickle down to the general public. This, in turn, has the potential to reduce the stigma that can lead to depression and anxiety. In sum, more research will lead to greater knowledge, which can turn the tide on the 'forgotten' people who may look well, but are very ill indeed. This is our hope and we will continue to try to be a small part of this shift by continuing our own research into long-term conditions and writing books so that the research isn't only available to the scientists and doctors, but also to those with the illnesses. Knowledge is power – it must be shared!

Final summary and conclusions

We sincerely hope that you have found this book helpful. Overall, if you take nothing else from this book, please know that there are many others out there with invisible illnesses. They may not have the same condition as you but there will be commonalities. These similarities will not necessarily be in terms of symptoms, although they may be. You may find that even if you have FMS and someone else suffers from migraines, the way in which symptoms have an impact on your lives is similar. Sharing your experiences and knowing that you are not alone in what you go through on a daily basis can help not just you but others too. Humans are at core social beasts, so do not feel afraid to reach out to others – they might just surprise you!

Useful addresses

Charities (UK)

Action for ME
PO Box 2778
Bristol BS1 9DJ
Tel.: 0845 123 2380 (lo-call) or 0117 927 9551 (9 a.m. to 5 p.m., Monday to Friday)
Website: www.actionforme.org.uk

Bladder and Bowel Foundation
SATRA Innovation Park
Rockingham Road
Kettering
Northants NN16 9JH
Tel.: 01536 533255 (general enquiries); 0845 345 0165 (helpline)
Website: www.bladderandbowelfoundation.org

British Tinnitus Association
Ground Floor, Unit 5
Acorn Business Park, Woodseats Close
Sheffield S8 0TB
Tel.: 0114 250 9922 (general enquiries); 0800 018 0527 (free of charge helpline from within UK only)
Website: www.tinnitus.org.uk

Fibromyalgia Association
Studio 3007, Mile End Mill
12 Seedhill Road
Paisley PA1 1JS
Tel.: 0844 887 2444 (general); 0844 826 9033 (10 a.m. to 2 p.m.); 0844 826 9022 (not for support calls)
Website: www.fmauk.org

IBS Network
Unit 1.12, SOAR Works
14 Knutton Road
Sheffield S5 9NU
Tel.: 0114 272 3253
Website: www.theibsnetwork.org

Mal de Débarquement Syndrome (MdDS)
Website: www.mdds.org.uk
An online-only support group for those with experience of this condition. See also the linked American online organization in this list.

ME Association
7 Apollo Office Court
Radclive Road
Gawcott
Bucks MK18 4DF
Tel.: 01280 818964 (9.30 a.m. to 3 p.m.); 0844 576 5326 (ME Connect helpline, 10 a.m. to 12 noon, 2 p.m. to 4 p.m., 7 p.m. to 9 p.m.)
Email (support): meconnect@meassociation.org.uk
Website: www.meassociation.org.uk

Ménière's Society
The Rookery
Surrey Hills Business Park
Sheephouse Lane, Wotton
Dorking
Surrey RH5 6QT
Tel.: 0845 120 2975 or 01306 876883
Website: www.menieres.org.uk

Migraine Action
Fourth Floor, 27 East Street
Leicester LE1 6NB
Tel.: 0116 275 8317 (10 a.m. to 4 p.m., Monday to Friday)
Website: www.migraine.org.uk

Migraine Trust
52–53 Russell Square
London WC1B 4HP
Tel.: 020 7631 6970
Website: www.migrainetrust.org

National Migraine Centre (registered national charity independent of the NHS)
22 Charterhouse Square
London EC1M 6DX
Tel.: 020 7251 3322
Website: www.migraineclinic.org.uk

Charities (USA)

CFIDS Association of America
PO Box 220398
Charlotte, NC 28222-0398
Tel: 001 704 365 2343
Website: www.solvecfs.org

MdDS Balance Disorder Foundation (all-volunteer non-profit foundation)
22406 Shannondell Drive
Audubon, PA 19403
Fax: 001 210 641 6077
Website: www.mddsfoundation.org
See also reference to the online group in the UK section of this list.

Complementary and alternative treatments

British Acupuncture Council
63 Jeddo Road
London W12 9HQ
Tel.: 020 8735 0400
Fax: 020 8735 0404
Website: www.acupuncture.org.uk

Complementary and Natural Healthcare Council
83 Victoria Street
London SW1H 0HW
Tel.: 020 3178 2199 (9.30 a.m. to 5.30 p.m., Monday to Friday)
Website: www.cnhc.org.uk

General Hypnotherapy Standards Council and General Hypnotherapy Register
PO Box 204
Lymington
Hants SO41 6WP
Website: www.general-hypnotherapy-register.com

The Hypnotherapy Association UK
14 Crown Street
Chorley
Lancs PR7 1DX
Tel.: 01257 262124
Website: www.thehypnotherapyassociation.co.uk

The National Hypnotherapy Society
19 Grafton Road
Worthing
West Sussex BN11 1QT
Tel.: 0870 850 3387
Website: www.nationalhypnotherapysociety.org

Miscellaneous

British Society of Hearing Aid Audiologists (BSHAA)
Website: www.bshaa.com
Audiologists in your local area can be located via this site.

Selected references

Afari, N., van der Meer, J., Bleijenberg, G., and Buchwald, D. (2005). 'Chronic fatigue syndrome in practice'. *Psychiatric Annals* 35(4):350–60.

Anderson, G., Maes, M., and Berk, M. (2012). 'Biological underpinnings of the commonalities in depression, somatization, and Chronic Fatigue Syndrome'. *Medical Hypotheses* 78: 752–56.

Beauregard, M. (2009). 'Effect of mind on brain activity: evidence from neuroimaging studies of psychotherapy and placebo effect'. *Nord J Psychiatry* 63: 5–16.

Buchwald, D. (1996). 'Fibromyalgia and chronic fatigue syndrome: similarities and differences'. *Rheumatic Disease Clinics of North America* 22: 219–43.

Cucchiara, B., Wolf, R. L., Nagae, L., et al. (2013). 'Migraine with aura is associated with an incomplete circle of Willis: results of a prospective observational study'. *PloS One* 8(7): e71007.

Deare, J., Zheng, Z., Xue, C., et al. (2013). 'Acupuncture for treating fibromyalgia'. *Cochrane Database of Systematic Reviews* 31(5): CD007070.

Delmar, C., Bøje, T., Dylmer, D., et al. (2005). 'Achieving harmony with oneself: Life with a chronic illness'. *Scandinavian Journal of Caring Sciences* 19: 204–12.

Donaldson, V. (2000). 'A clinical study of visualization on depressed white blood cell count in medical patients'. *Applied Psychophysiology and Biofeedback* 25(2), 230–35.

Fluge, Ø., Bruland, O., Risa, K., et al. (2011). 'Benefit from B-lymphocyte depletion using the anti-CD20 antibody rituximab in chronic fatigue syndrome. A double-blind and placebo-controlled study'. *PloS One* 6(10): e26358.

Gholamrezaei, A., Ardestani, S. K., and Emami, M. H. (2006). 'Where does hypnotherapy stand in the management of irritable bowel syndrome? A systematic review'. *Journal of Alternative and Complementary Medicine* 12(6): 517–27.

Gonsalkorale, W. (2006). 'Gut-directed hypnotherapy: the Manchester approach for treatment of irritable bowel syndrome'. *International Journal of Clinical and Experimental Hypnosis* 54(1): 27–50.

Gotts, Z., Deary, V., Newton, J., et al. (2013). 'Are there sleep-specific phenotypes in patients with chronic fatigue syndrome? A cross-sectional polysomnography analysis'. *BMJ* 3(6): e002999.

Grossman, P., Niemann, L., Schmidt, S., and Walach, H. (2004). 'Mindfulness-based stress reduction and health benefits: a meta-analysis'. *Journal of Psychosomatic Research* 57(1): 35–43.

Hackshaw, K., Rodriguez-Saona, L., Plans, M., et al. (2013). 'A bloodspot-based diagnostic test for fibromyalgia syndrome and related disorders'. *Analyst* 138(16): 4453–62.

Jason, L., Boulton, A., Porter, N. S., et al. (2010). 'Classification of Myalgic Encephalomyelitis/Chronic Fatigue Syndrome by types of fatigue'. *Behavioral Medicine* 36(1): 24–31.

Jason, L., Taylor, R., and Kennedy, C. (2000). 'Chronic fatigue syndrome, fibromyalgia, and multiple chemical sensitivities in a community-based sample of persons with chronic fatigue syndrome-like symptoms'. *Psychosomatic Medicine* 62(5): 655–63.

Kiecolt-Glaser, J., McGuire, L., Robles, T., and Glaser, R. (2002). 'Psychoneuroimmunology: psychological influences on immune function and health'. *Journal of Consulting and Clinical Psychology* 70(3): 537–47.

Lewis, S., Cooper, C., and Bennett, D. (1994). Psychosocial factors and chronic fatigue syndrome. *Psychological Medicine* 24(3): 661–71.

Moss-Morris, R., and Spence, M. (2006). 'To "lump" or "split" the functional somatic syndromes: can infectious and emotional risk factors differentiate between the onset of chronic fatigue syndrome and irritable bowel syndrome?' *Psychosomatic Medicine* 68:, 463–9.

Paquette, V., Levesque, J., Mensour, B., et al. (2003). 'Change the mind and you change the brain: effects of cognitive–behavioral therapy on the neural correlates of spider phobia'. *NeuroImage* 18: 401–9

Parker, A., Wessely, S., and Cleare, A. (2001). 'The neuroendocrinology of chronic fatigue syndrome and fibromyalgia'. *Psychological Medicine* 31(8): 1331–45.

Parker White, C., and White, M. B. (2011) 'Sleep problems and fatigue in chronically ill women'. *Behavioral Sleep Medicine* 9(3): 144–61.

Saad, M., and de Medeiros, R. (2013). 'Complementary therapies for fibromyalgia syndrome: a rational approach'. *Current Pain and Headache Reports* 17(8): 1–8.

Salas, R., and Kwan, A. (2012) 'The real burden of restless legs syndrome: clinical and economic outcomes'. *American Journal of Managed Care* 18(9 suppl): S207–12.

Tillisch, K., Labus, J., Kilpatrick, L., et al. (2013). 'Consumption of fermented milk product with probiotic modulates brain activity'. *Gastroenterology* 144(7): 1394–401.

Van Hoof, E. (2009) 'The doctor–patient relationship in chronic fatigue syndrome: survey of patient perspectives'. *Quality in Primary Care* 17: 263–70.

Wolfe, F., Smythe, J. A., Yunus, M. B., et al. (1990). 'The American College of Rheumatology 1990 Criteria for the Classification of Fibromyalgia: Report of the Multicenter Criteria Committee'. *Arthritis and Rheumatism* 36: 160–72.

Wysenbeek, A., Shapira, Y., and Leibovici, L. (1991). 'Primary fibromyalgia and the chronic fatigue syndrome'. *Rheumatology International* 10(6): 227–9.

Further reading

Beauregard, M. (2013). *Brain Wars: The Scientific Battle Over the Existence of the Mind and the Proof That Will Change the Way We Live Our Lives.* New York: HarperOne.

Carruthers, B., Jain, A., de Meirleir, K., et al. (2003). 'Myalgic encephalo-myelitis/chronic fatigue syndrome: clinical working case definition, diagnostic and treatment protocols'. *Journal of Chronic Fatigue Syndrome* 11(1): 7–36.

Clark, B. C., and Quick, A. (2011). 'Exploring the pathophysiology of mal de debarquement'. *Journal of Neurology* 258(6): 1166–8.

Diener, H., Dodick, D., Goadsby, P., Lipton, R, Olesen, J., and Silberstein, S. (2012). 'Chronic migraine: classification, characteristics and treatment'. *Nature Reviews. Neurology* 8(3): 162–71.

Dispenza, J. (2009). *Evolve Your Brain: The Science of Changing Your Mind.* Deerfield Beach, Florida: Health Communications.

Evans, P., Hucklebridge, F., and Clow, A. (2000). *Mind, Immunity and Health; the Science of Psychoneuroimmunology.* London: Free Association Books.

Häuser, W., Thieme, K., and Turk, D. (2010). 'Guidelines on the management of fibromyalgia syndrome: a systematic review'. *European Journal of Pain* 14(1): 5–10.

Kendall-Tackett, K. (ed.) *The Psychoneuroimmunology of Chronic Disease. Exploring the Links between Inflammation, Stress and Illness.* (2010). Washington, DC: American Psychological Association.

Syed, I., and Aldren, C. (2012). 'Ménière's disease: an evidence based approach to assessment and management'. *International Journal of Clinical Practice* 66(2): 166–70.

Yoon, S., Grundmann, O., Koepp, L., and Farrell, L. (2011). 'Management of irritable bowel syndrome (IBS) in adults: conventional and complementary/alternative approaches'. *Alternative Medicine Review*: 16(2): 134–51.

Index